Refractory Technology

Fundamentals and Applications

Refractory Technology

Fundamentals and Applications

Ritwik Sarkar

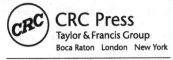

CRC Press
Taylor & Francis Group
Boca Raton London New York

CRC Press is an imprint of the
Taylor & Francis Group, an **informa** business

CRC Press
Taylor & Francis Group
6000 Broken Sound Parkway NW, Suite 300
Boca Raton, FL 33487-2742

First issued in paperback 2020

ISBN 13: 978-0-367-57429-1 (pbk)
ISBN 13: 978-1-4987-5425-5 (hbk)

Version Date: 20160822

Visit the Taylor & Francis Web site at
http://www.taylorandfrancis.com

and the CRC Press Web site at
http://www.crcpress.com

*Dedicated to my
Teachers,
Parents, and
Family*

———————————

Contents

List of Figures

List of Tables

Preface

CERAMIC MATERIALS HAVE BEEN part of the development of human society from its very beginning. Ceramic technology is one of the most ancient technologies; it is more than 24,000 years old and at the same time is the most modern, dynamically developing, and diverse field. The ever-increasing application of ceramics in different areas of space-age technology has made it an area of strategic importance. Among the various classes of ceramics, refractories are the materials possessing chemical and physical properties that make them suitable for structures or as components of the systems that are exposed to high temperatures.

The use of refractory has started since the invention of fire by humans and its controlled use. In the beginning, people started using clayey mass as a refractory to control the fire. In the initial stage of the metal age, crucible/pot-shaped natural rocks were used to soften and sharpen the weapons and primitive tools. With the ushering in of industrial revolution in eighteenth and nineteenth century, the concept of refractory technology underwent a change and new refractory materials other than naturally occurring clayey mass began to be used in different new furnaces and kilns. This period can be considered as the beginning point of the modern refractory technology. Many of the scientific and technological discoveries and advancements would not have taken place if the progress in refractory did not happen. But for a common man, refractories remained just a site for developing material required for high-temperature processing where metals cannot be used.

The operating environment for refractories is becoming increasingly severe with time. The rise in temperatures of operation, greater productivity, rapid thermal fluctuations, extremely corrosive environments, heavier loads, and extended service life and environmental constrictions have placed greater demand for the production of refractory products of superior quality. Hence for every specific application area, different classes of refractories with specific properties to withstand those environments are essential. Accordingly, various types of refractories have evolved over time.

Refractories need to prove their performances practically at the industrial conditions and scales. So it is essential for a refractory engineer to understand the concept of refractory, its basics and fundamentals, raw materials used, manufacturing methods, and properties of each of the refractories used in the different areas of different high-temperature processing. Also the interactions of the refractories with other materials, present in them as impurities or encountered during use at the user industry, are important. These interactions affect the properties and performance of the refractories. So a detailed understanding of these interactions is essential. But, unfortunately, the books available on refractory are extremely low to handle such a vivid industrial product. Hence, an up-to-date book covering these areas is essential to the refractory global community.

This book, *Refractory Technology: Fundamentals and Applications*, has been written to fill the scarcity of a complete book on refractory and also with an emphasis on fundamentals and applications of refractory materials. Chapter 1 provides a detailed introduction to refractory materials with a historical preview and current status. Chapter 2 deals with the classifications. Different types of classifications used in various refractory and user industries are covered with a brief introduction to each class of refractories. Chapters 3 and 4 deal with the properties of refractories and their testing methods. Properties are also classified as per their nature, such as physical, mechanical, thermal, thermo-mechanical, among others, and each individual property is discussed. Details of the testing methods of each of the individual properties of the refractories are described with relevant parameters for better understanding and information. Also, an introduction to standard specifications, as applied in different corners of the world, is incorporated in Chapter 4 to have a feeling of actual practice.

Chapters 5 through 12 deal with the common and individual types of refractories used in various industries. Common items like raw materials, manufacturing methods, subclassifications used in that particular refractory, and properties and applications are provided for silica, alumina, fireclay, magnesia, doloma, magnesia-carbon, and chrome containing refractories. Moreover, the effect of impurities, which these refractories encounter during their application, has also been discussed with the necessary phase diagrams for a better understanding of the refractory in a particular chemical environment. However, binary phase diagrams are only mentioned here as the higher number of components may complicate the understanding. Chapter 12 describes some special refractory materials that are highly useful for the incorporation of a certain specific property but used in a limited extent mainly due to their availability and cost.

Unshaped refractory is covered in Chapter 13. As on today, literature and books available on refractories have completely separated the shaped and unshaped materials. In this book, they are incorporated together to have the idea of unshaped materials in parallel with the shaped ones. Though unshaped refractory has started its commercial success more than 100 years ago, it has strongly developed and is being widely used in the last 30 or so years. Evolving from simple mixes of materials with different sizes, today's unshaped refractory is based on complex and advanced formulations with multiple additives, applied by different advanced techniques and resulting in better performances with enhanced life. Chapter 13 includes classification of unshaped refractories, details of various types of materials, and additives used in making them and brief details of each type of unshaped refractories along with the main application areas.

Ritwik Sarkar

Author

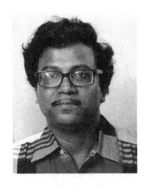

Ritwik Sarkar has been an associate professor in the Department of Ceramic Engineering, National Institute of Technology, Rourkela, India, since 2009. He completed his degree in ceramic technology from the University of Calcutta in 1993, postgraduate degree in ceramic engineering from the Banaras Hindu University (BHU) in 1995, and a PhD from Jadavpur University in 2003, all from India.

Before his current profession, Dr. Sarkar worked as General Manager—Technology, IFGL Refractories Ltd., India during 2008–2009. He has also worked as a scientist in the Central Glass and Ceramic Research Institute, India, 2001–2008, in the Research and Consultancy Directorate, ACC Ltd., Thane, India during 1999–2001 and at H & R Johnson (I) Ltd., Thane in 1995. He was a postdoctoral research fellow in the Institute of Ceramic Components in Mechanical Engineering (IKKM), Rheinisch-Westfälische Technische Hochschule (RWTH), Aachen, Germany, with DAAD (German Academic Exchange Service) Fellowship, during 2003–2004.

Dr. Sarkar's current areas of interest and research works include the development of refractory aggregates, unshaped and castable refractories, use of nanocarbon in carbon containing refractories, spinel-based ceramics, machinable bioceramics, and solid waste utilization. A life member of The Indian Ceramic Society and the Indian Institute of Ceramics, Dr. Sarkar is the assistant editor of *IRMA* (Indian Refractory Makers' Association) *Journal* and a reviewer of many prestigious research journals. He has more than 130 research publications and 9 patents to his credit.

Dr. Sarkar has received gold medals from BHU and Jawaharlal Nehru Memorial Fund's award for his academic excellence and the Young Scientist Award, the Ganpule Award, and the Deokaran Award from the Indian Ceramic Society for his scientific and research contributions to ceramic science and engineering.

CHAPTER 1

Introduction to Refractory

1.1 INTRODUCTION

Ceramic materials have been closely related to the development of human society from its very beginning. Ceramic technology is one of the most ancient of the technologies; it is more than 24,000 years old and at the same time is the most modern, dynamically developing, and diverse field. The ever-increasing applications of ceramics in different areas of space-age technology have made it a field of strategic importance too. Ceramic materials in the form of cement, glasses, enamels, porcelains, claywares, etc. have responded to the fundamental human needs by providing building materials for shelter, pots for cooking and storage and many other aspects. Among the different classes of ceramics, refractories are the materials that can withstand high temperature under a high load. In other words, refractories are heat-resistant materials that constitute the linings for high-temperature furnaces and reactors and other processing units. They are resistant to thermal stress and other thermal energy–related physical phenomena, in addition to withstanding mechanical loads and shocks, resisting abrasion and wear of the frictional forces and corrosion by chemical agents. And all these phenomena occur simultaneously in an environment of the different partial pressure of oxygen at high temperatures. Refractories act as the "backbone of industry" because they are essentially required to support the production of all the basic and essential commodities manufactured at high temperatures, like iron and steel, aluminum, copper, cement, glass, chemicals and petrochemicals, ceramics, etc.

Hence, it is clear that refractories are required for withstanding the heat and any process associated with high temperature require refractories. Table 1.1 shows different high-temperature industries and the associated temperature of processing. All these high-temperature processing industries require refractories. Among all the different industries, the consumption of refractories varies, and Figure 1.1 shows the main refractory consuming industries with the percentage consumption to the total refractory produced.

As iron and steel products are the primary materials that human civilization requires in the present day, the demand for iron and steel is also high compared to any other material. Hence, the consumption of refractories for these industries is also high, which is nearly three-fourths

TABLE 1.1   Some High Temperature Industrial Processes

Industries	Range of Temperatures (°C)
Industrial drying	50–300
Petrochemical industries	100–1100
Hydroxide calcination	400–800
Glass annealing	400–800
Carbon combustion	400–900
Steam boiler	400–1000
Sulfide ore roasting	400–1200
Heat treatment and annealing of metals	500–1300
Aluminum and magnesium	800–1100
Carbonate calcining	800–1300
Sulfate decomposition	800–1400
Foundry industry and rolling mills	900–1400
Salt glazing of conventional ceramics	1000–1300
Fusion process	1000–2200
White ware industries	1100–1500
Glass making	1300–1500
Phosphate decompose	1300–1700
Iron making and steel making	1300–1800
Baking of carbon	1300–1800
Sintering of oxides	1300–1800
Refractories	1300–1850
Portland cement	1350–1700
Sintering of carbides	1500–1900
Sintering of carbide	1500–2000
SiC industries	1800–2200
Refractory metals	1900–2200

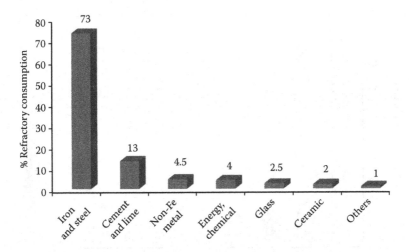

FIGURE 1.1   Industry wise global refractory consumption (in percent).

of the total refractory manufactured. Therefore, as iron and steel industry drives the developments of the refractory industries, the developmental activities in refractories have mostly followed the requirements generated by the advancements in the iron and steel industries.

The iron and steel industry is growing phenomenally, and China has taken the lead role in both manufacturing and consumption of iron and steel. Figures 1.2 and 1.3 show the countries that are principal iron and steel manufacturers and consumers. Currently, the global crude steel production is about 1.6 billion tons and China alone produces close to 50% of

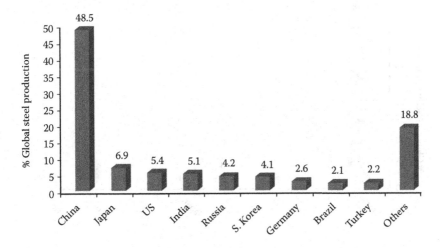

FIGURE 1.2   Major iron and steel producing countries.

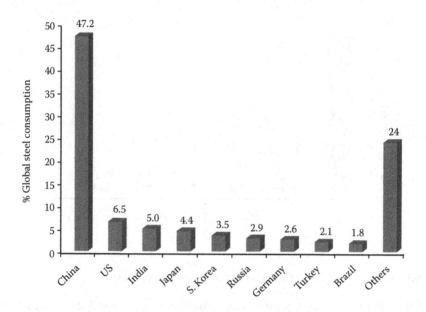

FIGURE 1.3   Major iron and steel consuming countries.

this quantity. As the refractory industries mainly follow the trend of the iron and steel industries, the largest producer of iron and steel, China, is the largest producer and consumer of refractories, followed by the other main iron and steel manufacturing countries. Globally, the total refractory production is about 38.6 million tons. Figure 1.4 shows the primary

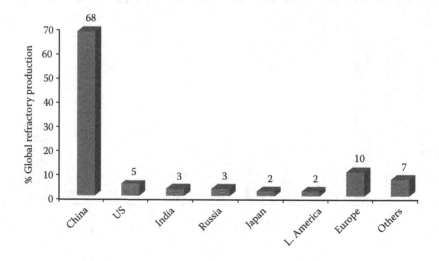

FIGURE 1.4   Major refractory producing countries.

refractory manufacturing countries with their percentage of share in the global refractory production.

1.2 DEFINITION

The word "refractory" originates from Latin word *refrāctārius*, which means stubborn or obstinate. In Webster's English dictionary, refractory is defined as a material that does not significantly deform or change chemically at high temperatures. Also in other classical dictionaries, refractories are defined as materials that are hard to work with and are especially resistant to heat and pressure.

As per ASTM C71 specification, refractories are defined as "non-metallic materials having those chemical and physical properties that make them applicable for structures, or as components of systems, that are exposed to environments above 1000°F (~811°K or 538°C)." And as per general understanding, refractories are non-metallic inorganic materials suitable for use at high temperatures in furnace construction. While their primary function is to resist the high temperatures under high load, they are also called on to resist other destructive influences during the heat processing, such as abrasion pressure, chemical attack, and rapid changes in temperature. In practical terms, refractories are the products used for any high-temperature processing to insulate the system, introduce erosion–corrosion–abrasion resistances against the process conditions, and are made mainly from non-metallic minerals. They are designed and processed in such a way that they become resistant to the corrosive and erosive action of hot gases, liquids, and solids at high temperatures in various types of kilns and furnaces.

While these definitions correctly identify the fundamental characteristics of refractories—their ability to provide containment of substances at high temperature—refractories comprise of a broad class of materials having the above characteristics to varying degrees, for varying periods of time, and under varying conditions of use. There are a wide variety of refractory compositions fabricated in a large range of shapes, sizes, and forms, which have been adapted to a wide variety of applications. The common denominator is that whenever a refractory is used, it will be subjected to high temperatures.

1.3 BASIC PROPERTY REQUIREMENTS

It is now clear that refractories are the industrial materials that are primarily required for any high-temperature processing and must have two very basic features, high temperature withstandability (high melting point) and high strength at high temperatures. Other than these two, the refractories need to have very low deformability against time at continuous high-temperature conditions, that is, refractories must have high creep resistances. Also, prolonged or repeated use at high temperature may cause some dimensional changes of the refractory due to internal structural adjustments, which may cause deviation from dimension accuracy and may result in failure of the refractories. Hence, very high volume stability even on prolonged use is essentially required.

Again, any high-temperature processing may involve some chemical reactions using various chemicals with varying acidity and basicity, and generation of liquids and gaseous products as reaction products of the processing. Hence, the refractories have to withstand such chemical environments and need to have excellent corrosion resistances. All the processes are needed with some input materials to produce the desired products. Hence, refractories are associated with the flow of the materials, both charge and product. Again these materials may be solid, liquid, or gas, either in a continuous fashion or a batch process having one entry side and one exit side (both the entry of raw materials and exit of reaction products may occur from the same side in a batch type of processing). Hence, refractories are affected by the movement of the materials and requiring excellent resistances against abrasion, erosion, and wear.

Excellent mechanical properties, especially strength, at elevated temperatures is necessary for refractories. Apart from these, some basic thermal properties are also important. Increase in the dimension of any materials with increasing temperature is an atomistic property (reversible thermal expansion). Now this increasing dimension with increasing temperature may cause a problem for the structural integrity of the refractory vessel. Different refractories with different expansion properties change in the overall dimensions of the refractory lining and may result in a huge thermal strain and crack. Hence, any refractory needs to have a lower thermal expansion property so that the thermal stress generated will be minimum. In addition, thermal conductivity is another important fundamental thermal property. The primary purpose of the use of a refractory is to insulate the high-temperature process from the low-temperature environment. Otherwise, heat will pass through resulting in an enormous requirement of thermal energy. Hence, lower thermal conductivity is preferable to reduce the heat loss and make the process economical. Again lower thermal conductivity in a very high-temperature process may produce a very high thermal gradient in the refractory surfaces, one facing the high temperature of the process and the other one facing the ambient atmosphere. This huge temperature gradient will produce a significant thermal strain, resulting in thermal shock and cracking of the refractory. So to have a high thermal shock resistance, the refractory again needs to pass on heat from the inner surface to outer one, hence, may require high thermal conductivity too.

Refractories as conventional ceramics are processed from granular/powdered materials (exactly opposite to any metal/glass product) and the presence of porosity (void) is inherent in them. The presence of porosity results in a poor strength and also results in weak resistances to corrosion, abrasion, and wear. Hence, porosity must be minimum for a strong and dense refractory. Similar to porosity, permeability is also detrimental to refractory. But porosity is desired for refractories that are used only for heat insulting purposes as the pores are filled up with static air, which is one of the best insulator and results in a high thermal efficiency of any high-temperature process.

For any application, the general requirements for a refractory material are as follows:

- It has to withstand high temperatures even under high load.

- It has to have high volume stability.

- It has to withstand sudden changes in temperature.

- It has to withstand the action of molten metal slag, glass, hot gases, etc.

- It has to withstand the abrasive/wear/erosive forces.

- It should have a low coefficient of thermal expansion.

- It should be able to conserve heat.

- It should not contaminate the product/process material.

1.4 HISTORY OF REFRACTORY DEVELOPMENT

The manufacturing process of a refractory is quite similar to the formation of basalt, a naturally occurring siliceous rock. Basalt forms from lava that flows out from volcanic eruptions under the natural geological forces of heat and pressure. Refractory production is somewhat a replication of this natural process where, in general, the naturally occurring (or synthetic) non-metallic mineral oxides (and some non-oxides in special cases) convert to refractory under the conditions of high heat and pressure mostly in solid state.

Since very ancient times, the developments in refractory technology follows the similar track of the developments of the ceramic and metal industries. Refractories are known to exist since the period of Bronze and Iron Ages, more than 10,000 years ago. In the early Bronze Age, a kind of pit kiln was used to fire the earthen wares, where green earthenwares were placed in a hole, dug into the ground for firing. The soil around the dug-out portion used to act a heat-/fire-resistant material, and the upper limit of such kilns was the decomposition temperature of those soil/clayey materials. Naturally, the cavities for the pit kilns were made in such an area where the soil is relatively more heat resistant, insulating and resistant to any crack formation on heating and breaking. In today's technical term, the refractories that were used for such firing are nothing but clay refractories.

With time, civilization entered the iron age when remarkable improvements in refractories were observed. Iron was produced by reducing iron ore with charcoal in a furnace at a temperature much higher than the pottery making temperatures. The furnace lining had to withstand not only the temperature but also the mechanical action and chemical corrosion of the process and wear of the charge and product materials. Natural stones (mostly silica containing), fire clays, and a mixture of charcoal and clay were the standard materials for furnace lining. Evidence of iron-making furnaces was found in Europe in the fourteenth century.

Study on the history of glassmaking depicts that the first perfect glass was made in coastal north Syria, Mesopotamia, or ancient Egypt way back in 3500 BC. In the modern history, evidence of glass pots, the refractory vessel for glass melting, were found in Salem, Massachusetts, in 1638. Fire bricks were reported to be manufactured in England in the seventeenth century and used to be transported to different countries for glass manufacturing. In the late eighteenth century, fire brick making was started in the United States.

Again if we look into the history of refractory making, it can be found that silica refractories were reported to be manufactured initially in South Wales, England, way back in 1842 and later in 1899 it was started in the Mount Union region of Pennsylvania in the United States. Magnesite refractories were initially started in Austria, Europe, around 1880 and in 1888 its manufacturing was started in Homestead, Pennsylvania.

The first reported application of dolomite lining was found during the invention of the process of phosphorous removal in Bessemer route of steel making by Sidney Gilchrist Thomas and his cousin Percy Gilchrist in 1878. Use of pure chrome refractories were started since 1896 and chrome-mag refractories were commenced in 1931 when it was found that the mix of chrome and magnesite had better tensile strength properties than the components alone and resulted in better thermal shock resistances. Direct bonded chrome-mag refractories were first launched in 1961. In modern days, the official record of the first use of unshaped refractory, as plastic mass, was found in 1914 by W. A. L. Schaefer. Electrofused cast refractories were invented in the mid-1920s while the inventors, H. Hood and G. S. Fulcher were studying the stubborn, glass-insoluble inclusion "stones."

Thus, the development of refractory has been happening with time, and new types or a combination of different refractory components are being studied, invented, and applied for the betterment of the user industry, resulting in a better quality product, productivity, longevity, and performances of the refractory lining.

1.5 SUMMARY

Among the various types of ceramics refractories are those materials that have excellent strength even at high temperatures.

Refractories consist of a broad class of materials (mostly oxides) having different types of characteristics to varying degrees at high temperatures, for varying periods of time, and under varying conditions of applications.

As per ASTM C71, refractories are "non-metallic materials having those chemical and physical properties that make them applicable for structures, or as components of systems, that are exposed to environments above 1000°F (811°K; 538°C)."

The basic properties that a refractory must have are the following:

- Ability to withstand high temperature
- High strength at high temperatures
- High creep resistance
- High volume stability
- Excellent corrosion resistance

- Resistance to wear, abrasion, and erosion

- Low thermal expansion

- High thermal shock resistance

- Thermal conductivity (low or high depending on properties of thermal shock and insulation)

- Density and porosity (depending on dense or insulating character requirements)

Refractory is an ancient technology, since the invention of fire. It is not a directly consumable product rather it is an ancillary industry. Refractories are a must for all the high-temperature operations. The industry grows along with the growth and requirement of the user industries. About 75% of the total refractory produced is used in iron and steel industry. The main steel manufacturing and consuming country, China, is the leading manufacturer of refractories.

QUESTIONS AND ASSIGNMENTS

1. What is a refractory?

2. What are the basic functions of a refractory material?

3. What are the main properties that a refractory must have?

4. Describe the functions of refractories that a high-temperature processing industry may require.

5. How has the growth of the refractory industry taken place?

BIBLIOGRAPHY

1. S. Musikant, *What Every Engineer Should Know About Ceramics*, Preface, Marcel Dekker Inc., New York, 1991.
2. W. W. Perkins, *Ceramics Glossary 1984*, The American Ceramic Society, Ohio, US, p. 91.
3. J. G. Hemrick, H. W. Hayden, P. Angelini, R. E. Moore, and W. L. Headrick, *Refractories for Industrial Processing: Opportunities for Improved Energy Efficiency*, Prepared for the DOE-EERE Industrial Technologies Program, January 2005.

4. J. Roberts, Outlook for refractory end markets to 2020, *Presented at the 57th International Colloquium on Refractories*, Aachen, Germany, September 24–25, 2014.
5. J. Roberts, Outlook for refractory end markets to 2020, *57th International Colloquium on Refractories*, 24–25 September, Aachen, Germany, 2014.
6. K. Sugita, Historical overview of refractory technology in the steel industry, Nippon Steel Technical Report, No 98, July 2008, pp. 8–17. http://www.nssmc.com/en/tech/report/nsc/pdf/n9803.pdf.
7. Refractory market—RHI AG, May 2015. http://www.rhi-ag.com/linkable blob/internet_en/4134/data/Unternehmenspraesentation-data.pdf.
8. A. H. Al-Shorman, Refractory ceramic through the ages: An archaeometric study on finds from Fenan, Jordan and other sites, doctoral thesis, Ruhr University, Bochum, October 2009.
9. *World Steel in Figures*, World Steel Association, Brussels, Belgium, 2014, ISBN 978-2-930069-73-9.

CHAPTER 2

Classifications of Refractories

2.1 INTRODUCTION

The wide variety of high-temperature processing across various industries demands diversity in the refractory materials. The diversity requirements may arise from application temperatures, atmospheric conditions that prevail during the processing, mechanical, thermal, chemical, abrading and wear conditions, and so on. In fact, many of the refractory materials have been developed to meet precisely certain service conditions of particular pyro-processing conditions. To meet this wide variety of application conditions, different classes of refractory materials are required and are being developed as time progresses. For example, the atmosphere of the processing condition demands a refractory of basic or acidic character, the temperature may be very high or low, some applications may require very strong and dense refractory, and in some cases, the requirement is to insulate the process.

This wide variety of application conditions in different industries is required to be well understood by the refractory manufacturers and developers, and they need to provide a variety of refractories suitable for each and every condition. This variety of refractories can be classified as per various groups/classes based on certain specific properties. These different categories of refractory classification with their detailed subclasses are described in this chapter. These different classes are based on the following:

1. Chemical nature: As per chemical nature refractories are classified as

    a. Acidic refractory

    b. Basic refractory

    c. Neutral refractory

2. Manufacturing method: The refractories are manufactured through different techniques or processing and as per that specific or special techniques used, the refractories are classified. For example

    a. Pressed and fired refractory

    b. Fused cast refractory

    c. Hand molded refractory

3. Physical form/shape: Classification is also important as per the physical form of the refractory, and the main subclasses are the following:

    a. Shaped refractory like bricks, having a definite shape and size during manufacturing and supply to the user industry

    b. Unshaped refractory like castables, which are well mixed granular masses and does not have any specific shape and dimension during manufacturing and supply to user industry

4. Porosity (insulating nature): The amount of porosity describes the dense (strong) or insulating character of a material. Refractories are classified as per porosity as

    a. Dense refractory

    b. Insulating refractory

5. Heat duty (application temperature): This classification is based on the maximum temperature that a refractory can withstand or indicates the maximum application temperature. The traditional nomenclatures are

    a. High heat duty

    b. Medium heat duty

    c. Low heat duty, etc.

6. Main constituent: Refractories are classified as per the principal chemical component (normally oxide) present in them and named accordingly. For example

   a. Silica refractory, when the main constituent is silica

   b. Alumina refractory, when the main constituent is alumina

7. Purity: Within the classification of the main constituent, depending on the percent (purity) of that constituent present, the refractories are further classified. For example

   a. 60% alumina brick (means major constituent of the brick is alumina and the amount of alumina present is 60%)

   b. 70% alumina brick

8. Special refractory: Refractories that do not come under the above broad classifications and typically used at a much reduced volume, only in special cases, such as

   a. Non-oxide containing refractory

   b. Zirconia refractory, etc.

The sections that follow review the primary classifications of refractories that are most common and commercially utilized, taking into account their main features related to their nomenclature and most typical applications.

2.2 CLASSIFICATION BASED ON CHEMICAL NATURE

Refractories are very commonly classified based on their chemical behavior, that is, how a refractory will behave in a particular environment. Chemical environments prevailing in the furnace or the processing conditions determine the most suitable refractory for such an application. As per the chemical nature (affinity) of any material, refractories are classified as acidic, basic, and neutral.

2.2.1 Acidic Refractories

Acidic refractories are those that are resistant to any acidic conditions like slag, fume, and gases at high temperatures. But they are readily attacked by any basic slag or environment. In the presence of any basic components, the acidic refractories react with it rapidly, causing a massive corrosion in the refractory lining and resulting in a very poor life of the lining.

These refractories are only used in areas where slag and atmosphere are acidic. Examples of acid refractories are as follows:

1. Silica (SiO_2)

2. Fireclay

Both the refractories contain silica as the main material and in any basic environment at high temperature, say in the steel ladles or burning zone of cement kilns, they will react and form various silicates. These silicate compounds have low melting points, and they further react with solid refractory structure, causing wear of refractory and drastic deterioration of refractory lining. Hence, any acidic refractory performs best in an acidic environment, say in glass melting tank applications, if other application criteria are met.

2.2.2 Neutral Refractories

Neutral refractories are chemically stable to both acids and bases and are used in areas where slag and atmosphere are either acidic or basic. Hence, these types of refractories are most commonly preferred. But many of the refractories that behave as neutral at low temperatures behave with some chemical affinity at high temperatures. Hence neutral refractory, useful for very high aggressive environments at high temperature, is rare.

The typical examples of these materials are as follows:

1. Carbon or graphite (most inert)

2. Alumina (Al_2O_3)

3. Chromia/chrome oxide (Cr_2O_3)

Out of these materials, graphite is the least reactive and is extensively used in metallurgical furnaces where the process of oxidation of carbon can be controlled. Alumina and chromia are stable at low temperatures but at high temperatures, they behave a little acidic in nature and react with very strong basic materials. Hence, at high temperatures, their chemical neutrality is no longer valid.

2.2.3 Basic Refractories

Basic refractories are those materials that are attacked by acidic components but stable against alkaline slags, dust, fumes, and environments at elevated temperatures. Since these refractories do not react with alkaline slags, they are of considerable importance in basic steel-making processes, non-ferrous metallurgical operations, and cement industries. The most common important basic refractories are the following:

1. Magnesia (MgO)

2. Doloma (CaO · MgO)

Basic refractories are never used in acidic conditions, say in glass melting tank, where they will be washed away very fast by forming low-melting silicates.

2.3 CLASSIFICATION BASED ON MANUFACTURING METHOD

Manufacturing methods of the refractories vary to attain definite shape, size, and specific properties. The nomenclature of the refractories is also done as per the different manufacturing techniques employed. The various subclasses of this classification are as follows.

2.3.1 Pressed and Fired (Sintered)

This is the most common and conventional type of refractory that is generally found. In this method, particles of different sizes (of various raw materials to get the proper refractory composition) are mixed and then pressed and fired to attain the desired shape and characteristics. Pressing pressure and firing temperatures are critical parameters and are fixed as per the constituents of the composition and targeted properties. The use of lower pressure and temperature results in a low strength and relatively porous (less dense) product.

2.3.2 Fused Cast

Fused cast refractories are important for many industries like glass, iron and steel, and aluminum, where the refractories are subjected to remain in contact with the liquid phase at high temperature for a prolonged period. They are also necessary for petrochemical and other related industries where the refractories are subject high wear, abrasion, erosion, and chemical attack. Fused cast refractories are manufactured by melting mixtures of oxide powders (for the desired composition) in an electric arc furnace (using carbon electrodes) at a temperature exceeding 2000°C and casting the melt in molds wherein it solidifies through annealing to reduce the generation of strain. These refractories are treated with oxygen while in the molten state to place the constituents in the most highly oxidized state. A contraction cavity is formed beneath the casting scar during cooling, and so the opposite surface of the casting scar is used as the working face of the refractory.

Compared to conventional refractories, fused cast products have a very dense and highly durable structure using stable mineral substances, and it shows particularly superior mechanical and chemical properties. Also, fusion and slow cooling produce large crystal sizes that reduce surface area for any chemical reaction and resulting in increased corrosion resistances. Low porosities restrict the ingress of corrosive liquids, and the smooth surface prevents the adhesion of slag. These refractories can resist high surface loads due to high heat compression strength. Again high thermal conductivity from dense structure results in a uniform heat distribution within the refractory, producing an uniform thermal condition. But as the process involved melting of refractory materials, enormous amount of heat is required to manufacture these refractories that affect the economy.

2.3.3 Hand Molded

These refractories are important for their critical shapes and sizes. Non-conventional, critical shapes, and dimensions in refractories are important for many special applications, like in coke ovens, glass tank furnace, etc. Pressing is a simple method for great productivity but pressing molds cannot produce intricate shapes as the releasing of the pressed shapes needs a simple design for higher productivity. Also, dimensions of the shape is also limited to pressing process as much bigger dimensions requires huge pressing capacity, which has certain technical limitations. Hence for forming a complicated shape or a large-sized refractory product before firing, hand molding (using techniques like hammering) is the easiest and simple process.

As hand-generated pressure is much lower than the pressing pressure, the amount of water used is about two to three times more than that required for pressing. Also, the green strength is lower for hand molded products. Hence, handling and drying of these types of refractories are relatively critical. Higher moisture content and less compaction pressure during shaping of these products produce relatively porous structure and high shrinkage on firing, and so the mold size needs to be adjusted accordingly.

2.3.4 Bonding

Most of the refractories are sintered; this means they have a ceramic bond in between the loose starting particles from which they have been prepared. Other than this sintering and ceramic bond, many bonds are also used for the refractories as per the composition and requirement.

Many of the refractories are chemically bonded. That means a different chemical bonding material is used, which is entirely different from the basic composition of the refractory, to create a secondary (chemical) bond between the particles to retain the shape and size, generate strength, and other properties. Mostly chemical bonding is used for those refractory systems that require a very high temperature to develop a direct sintering (ceramic) bond. The addition of a secondary phase may form a liquid (or reacts and melts) and creates a bonding between the particles of the primary refractory particles. But the high-temperature properties of the refractory get affected.

Also, tar/pitch/resin bonding is common for refractories containing carbon in the composition at a considerable amount. Carbon particles, which are having very strong atomic bonding in-between themselves and are very fine, when present in between the refractory oxide particles, do not allow the refractory for mass transfer and sintering even at high temperatures. Hence, for carbon containing systems, carbon based bonding especially, liquid carbonaceous materials are used as bonding material that can polymerize and form a three-dimensional carbon-based network structure. This three-dimensional network can hold the whole refractory structure or particles, even at high temperatures and provide strength.

2.4 PHYSICAL FORM OR SHAPE

As per the physical form of the refractory, they are classified as per the following.

2.4.1 Shaped

These types of refractories have fixed size and shapes. Shaped refractories are the most common and conventional ones. Shapes may be standard ones and special types. Standard shapes are those products whose shape and dimensions are common and accepted by most of the refractory manufacturers and users. Standard-shaped bricks have dimensions that conform to most of the refractory manufacturers and are applicable to kilns and furnaces of the same type. Standard shapes are usually required in vast quantities to construct a kiln or furnace.

On the other hand, special shapes are specially made for particular kilns or furnaces, with very specific shape and dimensions and are generally required only in limited quantities. Standard-shaped refractories are always machine-pressed and thus have uniformity of properties. Special shapes are usually hand molded and are generally associated with slight variation in properties.

2.4.2 Unshaped

Unshaped refractories are those which are made in loose granular condition and do not have any particular shape and size while they are transported to the user industry. The shape and size are given as per the requirement of the particular application by making it a flowable or shapeable mass and applying the same to the required area by casting, ramming, troweling, and gunning. As a very big and single structure can be made from these materials, they are also called monolithic (in Latin, *mono* means single and *lithus* means structure).

2.5 POROSITY (INSULATING)

Porosity differentiates the refractories into two major classes.

2.5.1 Dense

Dense refractories are those which have a very low porosity and are highly sintered to attain maximum possible packing and densification. Higher densification (lower porosity) comes from more and more contact in-between the particles due to a greater extent of packing (compaction/pressing) and sintering. A greater degree of grain-to-grain contact and sintering will produce greater strength. Hence, the dense refractory shows improved mechanical properties, higher resistances against corrosion, abrasion, wear and erosion, and increased thermal conductivity. Conventionally, refractories having porosity below 45% are termed as dense refractories.

2.5.2 Insulating

Any high-temperature processing requires a significant amount of thermal energy. And in most of the cases, the energy requirement for the actual process is much lower than the total energy consumed. This is due to the enormous amount of energy loss mainly through the walls of the processing container (that is, the refractories) into the atmosphere. And the higher the temperature of processing, the chance of heat loss is more.

To reduce the energy escaping from the process, a special kind of refractory lining material for the processing vessel is required, which is called insulating refractory. The primary function of the insulating refractory is to prevent or reduce the rate of heat flow (heat loss) through the walls of the furnaces. These refractories need to withstand the high temperature of its application and simultaneously need to be insulating (low thermal conductivity). Such requirements can be achieved by incorporation of porosity in the refractory body, which are actually small air pockets. Air is having very low heat conductivity, hence the more the porosity, the more will be the insulating character of the refractory. Generally, refractories having a porosity more than 45% are called insulating refractories. Small and uniformly distributed pores with a higher amount of porosity result in better quality of insulating character.

2.6 SUMMARY

The classification of refractories is done as per various parameters.

The most common parameters are chemical nature, manufacturing method, physical form, porosity, heat duty, main constituent, purity, among others.

As per chemical nature, they are acidic (silica), basic (magnesia), and neutral (alumina) types.

As per manufacturing methods, refractories are classified as pressed and sintered, fused cast, hand molded, chemically bonded, etc.

According to physical form, the refractories are shaped and unshaped (monolithic) types.

As per heat duty, refractory types are super heat duty, high heat duty, medium heat duty, and low heat duty.

As per main constituents, refractories are classified as silica refractories, alumina refractories, fireclay refractories, magnesia refractories, etc. In the commercial world and manufacturing, mostly refractories are classified as per this classification.

Classification based on purity of the main constituent (90% or 80%) is a subclass of the above types.

As per porosity, refractories are dense (porosity <45%) and insulating (porosity >45%).

QUESTIONS AND ASSIGNMENTS

1. Why do we need a classification of refractories?

2. What do you understand by classification of refractories?

3. What are the different classification parameters of refractories?

4. Describe in detail the classification of refractories as per chemical nature.

5. Write in detail about the classification of refractories based on manufacturing methods.

6. Describe the porosity-based classification of refractories.

BIBLIOGRAPHY

1. C. A. Schacht, *Refractories Handbook*, CRC Press, Boca Raton, FL, 2004.
2. J. H. Chesters, *Refractories—Production and Properties*, Woodhead Publishing Ltd., Cambridge, UK, 2006.
3. P. P. Budnikov, *The Technology of Ceramics and Refractories*, 4th edn., translated by E. Arnold, *Scripta Technica*, The MIT Press, Cambridge, MA, 2003.
4. *Harbison-Walker Handbook of Refractory Practice*, Harbison-Walker, PA, 2005.
5. C. Barry Carter and M. Grant Norton, *Ceramic Materials: Science and Engineering*, Springer Science Business Media, New York, 2013.
6. S. C. Carniglia and G. L. Barna, *Handbook of Industrial Refractories Technology: Principles, Types, Properties, and Applications*, Noyes Publications, Saddle River, New Jersey, 1992.
7. A. R. Chesti, *Refractories: Manufacture, Properties and Applications*, Prentice-Hall of India, New Delhi, India, 1986.

CHAPTER 3

Idea of Properties

3.1 INTRODUCTION

Understanding the properties of refractory materials is important for gaining knowledge on the subject that will aid in the selection of refractories for a particular application and the development, improvement, and quality control of the refractories. Refractories, by definition, are those materials that can resist heat, corrosion of solids, liquids, and gaseous materials, abrasion and thermal shock and can withstand different degrees of mechanical stress and strain at various temperatures. The compositional adjustments are used in the design of different refractories and they are manufactured to optimize the properties that are appropriate for their applications in particular environments.

The quality of any refractory and its suitability for any specific application environment do not depend on any specific property. Rather, it is a combination of different properties that finally decides whether that particular refractory is suitable for any specific environment or not. Hence, a set of properties are important for a refractory. The set of properties required for a refractory may change from one application to another and the refractories that satisfy all the required property criteria are the most suitable for such applications.

There may be different groups of properties that are important for a refractory, and the most common groups of their detailed individual description are given below. Other than the common types of properties like physical, mechanical, and thermal, certain specific properties are also measured for refractories. These refractory-specific properties are also described separately at the end of the chapter.

3.2 PHYSICAL PROPERTIES

Properties that are easily measurable, whose values represent the state of a physical system, and the measurement processes do not change the identity of the material are called physical properties. In the measurement of physical properties, there should not be any chemical change or mechanical breakdown of the sample, and the physical form should remain intact. Physical properties can be used to characterize mixtures as well as pure substances. The changes in the physical properties of a system can be used to describe its transformations or evolutions between its momentary states.

Hence, by definition, physical property is a characteristic of a substance that can be observed or measured without changing its identity. All of the senses can be used to observe the physical properties like color, shape, size, etc. Mass, volume, and density are physical properties. Changing the mass or volume of a substance does not change the substance's identity. The state of matter that describes the physical form of the matter is also a physical property.

For refractories, the main physical properties measured are as follows.

3.2.1 Apparent Porosity, Total Porosity, and Bulk Density

The primary difference in manufacturing a metal or glass product and a ceramic product is their processing techniques. Any metal or glass item is made from a material that was in liquid state and processed to a solid state with specific shape and size. The formation of the liquid phase is beneficial as it is free from any air or void space (porosity) inside it, unless and otherwise it is entrapped during processing. But refractories and ceramics are made from loose granular mass having different sized particles and then firing it to a high temperature without or with a little liquid phase formation. Particularly for refractories, the liquid phase formation is nearly negligible (other than fused cast products) as that liquid phase will limit the high-temperature properties and applications of the refractory by a drastic reduction in hot strength. Hence the refractories are sintered in nearly solid state conditions, and the gap between the particles present at green condition (filled with air) are not completely removed (only reduced in size and total volume) even after firing/sintering.

Hence, refractories are not free from air pockets or voids, which in a solid mass are technically termed as "porosity." The porosity of a material is defined as the ratio of its pore volume to its bulk volume. The amount, size, and distribution of porosity control many of the refractory properties and also dictate the suitability of that refractory for a targeted application. Hence, it is important to measure the amount of porosity present in any refractory.

Porosities can be of two different types: open porosity and closed porosity. As the refractory surfaces are facing all the criticality of the application environment, the porosity present in the surface is most important, and its determination is essential. These surface porosities are called "apparent porosity." The apparent porosity is the ratio of the volume of the open (surface) pores, into which a liquid can penetrate, to that of the total volume of the sample, expressed as a percentage. This is an important property, especially where the refractory is in contact with molten charge and slag. A low apparent porosity is desirable since it would prevent easy penetration of any liquid into the refractory. Again, pore size and continuity of pores are important as they influence the behavior of the refractory against the molten material. Connectivity of pores is dangerous as it helps the liquid to penetrate into the interior of the refractory and cause the drastic deterioration. A large number of small pores is preferable compared to an equivalent volume of large pores from strength and chemical attack points of view. Apparent porosity (AP) is calculated as per the formula

$$\text{AP in } \% = \frac{(W-D)100}{W-S},$$

where D = weight of the dried sample, S = suspended the weight of the sample when immersed in liquid, and W = soaked weight, that is, the weight of the sample containing liquid in the surface pores or open pores but not in the free surfaces.

Closed porosities are those pores that are not visible unless the sample is broken. There is no direct method to view and measure them. They are closed from all the sides and very important for the thermal conductivity, strength, bulk weight of the samples, etc. Summation of closed and open porosities gives the value of total porosity.

Increase in porosity results in the following:

1. Poor conductivity: Pores or voids spaces are filled up with static air, and air has very low thermal conductivity. Hence the overall conductivity decreases. A refractory behaves like an insulating material at a very high level of porosity values.

2. Higher resistance against thermal fluctuation: As the pores are open space, they can accommodate the sudden expansions resulting in

from the thermal expansion property of sudden thermal fluctuations. Hence, strain generation will be less.

3. Poor strength: Higher porosity means less number of particles in contact, hence less resistance against any load and poor strength.

4. Poor resistance to abrasion, erosion, and wear.

5. Poor resistance to any chemical attack as the area for any reaction will increase due to the increased pore surfaces and easy penetration of corrosive liquids and gases.

6. High permeability: Higher porosity increases the chance of pore coalescence and pore connectivity resulting in higher permeability for any fluid through refractory.

Density is one of the most fundamental physical properties of any material. It is defined as the ratio of any shape's mass to its volume. As most of the designs are limited by either their size and or weight, density is an important consideration in many calculations. Now, the refractories have porosity within it, so the density is lower than their actual material's density. The presence of air pockets or voids or pores reduces the mass of the refractory. This reduced mass results in a decreased density of the refractory. The reduced density is required to be measured to get the idea of the total amount of refractory needed for a particular lining volume and overall weight calculation of the lining that will be present at the foundation of any furnace. This reduced density value that is useful for the refractories, containing some amount pores in it, is called "bulk density." It is defined as the weight per unit bulk volume of refractory, which also considers the volume of the pores. This bulk density indicates the actual densification of the material and gives an idea of the strength development and other related properties. Obviously, this density is lower than the true density of the material and the higher the amount of porosity, the lower will be the bulk density values. Bulk density (BD) is calculated as per the formula

$$BD = \frac{D\rho}{W - S},$$

where D = weight of the dried sample, S = suspended the weight of the sample when immersed in liquid, W = soaked weight, that is, the weight of the sample containing liquid in the surface or open pores but not on the free surfaces, and ρ = density of the liquid used for immersion at the test temperature.

3.2.2 Specific Gravity

The specific gravity is the ratio between the ideal density of an object (without any pore) and that of a reference substance at the same test conditions. Usually, the reference substance is water. This is also termed as true density that is the density of any material having no porosity. Simply put, specific gravity values indicate whether an object will sink or float or be a heavier or a lighter object. The specific gravity has no units because the units of the numerator and the denominator are the same, and so they just cancel out each other. Specific gravity varies with temperature and pressure, and so both the reference and test samples are to be compared at the same temperature and pressure conditions or otherwise, the specific gravity values are to be corrected for a standard reference temperature and pressure. Specific gravity and bulk density values will match when the total porosity value is "zero." For refractories, materials with very high specific gravity are not preferred as high specific gravity means higher amount of material for a fixed volume; so consumption of refractory material for lining a fixed dimension will be higher and total load (both weight and thermal load) of the lining will be higher with increased cost. Specific gravity values of some common refractory materials are given in Table 3.1.

3.2.3 Firing Shrinkage

This is the dimensional change that a refractory shape may have due to firing. As this property evaluation requires only the measurement of the

TABLE 3.1 Specific Gravity Values of Some Common Refractory Materials

Name	Specific Gravity
Alumina (corundum), Al_2O_3	3.99
Silica (quartz), SiO_2	2.65
Silica (cristobalite), SiO_2	2.32
Silica (tridymite), SiO_2	2.28
Magnesia, MgO	3.58
Iron oxide, Fe_2O_3	5.24
Zirconia, ZrO_2	6.1
Chrome oxide, Cr_2O_3	5.22
Lime, CaO	3.34
Mullite, $3Al_2O_3 \, 2SiO_2$	3.16
Spinel, $MgO \, Al_2O_3$	3.58
Silicon carbide, SiC	3.21
Graphite	2.2

dimension of the samples before and after firing, it is considered as a physical property. Shrinkage value is dependent on many parameters, the important ones are composition, firing temperature, soaking (dwelling) time, shaping pressure, etc. This property is more important for the refractory manufacturer than that of the user, as the manufacturer needs to adjust the unfired dimension and mold dimensions (as per the shrinkage value) to get the desired fired dimensions. Shrinkage, which is dimensional contraction during heat treatment (also during drying), occurs mainly due to removal (and reduction) of the pores (and pore volume) from the sample. Very high shrinkage values are not desirable due to the risk of warpages (non-flatness) or cracking of the sample during shrinking process. For situations where high shrinkage value may appear due to wide difference between unfired (dried) density and fired density, different or better shaping or compaction method must be introduced to reduce the shrinkage values.

Also, there are cases where expansion occurs during firing. This is due to some volume expansive reactions among the reactant phases (present in the composition) during firing or due to phase transformations of the reactant or product phases. This expansion also needs to be taken care similar to that of shrinkage. Shrinkage is calculated as per the formula

$$\text{Percent linear shrinkage} = \frac{(L_f - L_i)100}{L_i}$$

where L_i is the initial length of the refractory before firing and L_f is the final length of the refractory after firing.

3.2.4 Permeability

The rate at which a fluid can pass through porous materials is termed as permeability. Refractories having a higher amount of connectivity of its pores have a higher permeability. Low permeable refractories are essential for applications where they are in contact with gases and liquids.

3.3 MECHANICAL PROPERTIES

The mechanical properties of a refractory material determine how it will react to the mechanical forces that are present in its application area. In application, refractories face varied mechanical conditions with varying degrees of intensity, as they may be under compression, bending, shear, and also sometimes partial tension and twisting. Moreover, the refractories face all these different conditions not separately, but all the mechanical actions are active simultaneously to varying extents at different portions in the same application environment. So a combined action of several types of mechanical forces is present to varying extents. The major mechanical properties that are commonly measured for refractories are detailed below.

3.3.1 Cold Crushing Strength

This property indicates the compressive strength of a refractory material at ambient conditions or room temperature. Refractories have to withstand the structural load that are thrust upon them, mainly from the load of the refractory lining or furnace and also the load of the charge material. This property reveals the idea of load-bearing capacity of a refractory. CCS measures the bond rupture strength of a material under compression, and it has an indirect relevance to refractory performance.

Though many refractory technologists are not willing to assign due importance to this property, as dense refractories do not fail simply due to load at cold condition, but this can be used to get some idea about the quality and predictable performance of the refractory. Cold crushing strength (CCS) can be used as one of the indicators of abrasion resistance. The higher the CCS of a material, the greater is the resistance to abrasion, corrosion, etc. In general, higher sintering and higher densification results in higher CCS values. CCS is generally calculated on a cubic sample as per the formula:

$$CCS = \frac{P}{A},$$

where P = compressive load at which the refractory sample disintegrates and A = the area on which load is applied. Figure 3.1 shows the schematic of the CCS measurement. Ceramics are brittle materials and have pre-existing cracks due to their processing techniques. So, the bigger the size of the sample, the higher is the chance of having a larger-sized crack; even from the same material processed under the same conditions. Hence, the obtained strength will be lower as the size of the sample increases. So, the sample size of any refractory needs to be specified for any mechanical testing.

3.3.2 Cold Modulus of Rupture

Modulus of rupture (MOR), bending strength, or flexural strength is an important mechanical property, especially for brittle materials, and it

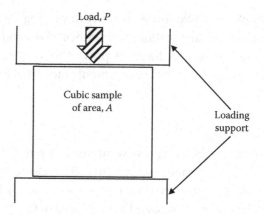

Load, *P*

Cubic sample
of area, *A*

Loading
support

FIGURE 3.1   Schematic of the CCS measurement.

measures the ability of the material to resist deformation under a bending load. When the measurement is done at ambient conditions or room
temperatures, then this is called as cold MOR. Here a bar-shaped specimen with circular or rectangular cross section is bent by applying the load
from the top and two supports from the bottom side until fracture. Most
commonly, two supporting points and one loading point test method are
used for refractories, called three points bending method. In some special cases, mostly for critical structural applications, two separate loading points are used along with two supporting points, called four-point
bending method. The flexural strength represents the highest stress
experienced within the material at its moment of rupture. Or in other
words, it is the ultimate strength of the failure of a bar-shaped material
by flexure equal to the bending moment of rupture divided by the section modulus of the bar. A schematic diagram of CMOR measurement is
shown in Figure 3.2. During bending under load, the sample extends to
the lower surface and contracts in dimension on the top surface. Hence,
the lower surface is under tension and the upper surface in under compression. As the ceramic materials are weak in tension, the crack of failure
under increasing load will start at the lower surface of the sample and then
extends till complete failure.

The important parameters for CMOR are loading rate (higher loading
rate will result in higher strength values), the size of the sample (greater
size will result in lower strength values), and porosity (higher porosity will
produce lower strength values). Flexural strength (σ) is calculated by the
formula:

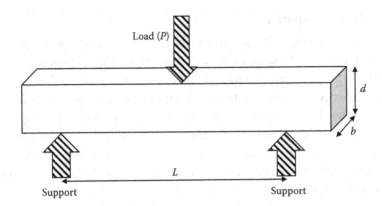

FIGURE 3.2   Schematic of the CMOR measurement for a rectangular bar sample.

$\sigma = 3PL / (2bd^2)$ in 3-point test of rectangular specimen

$\sigma = PL / (\pi r^3)$ in 3-point test of round specimen

$\sigma = 3Pa / (bd^2)$ in 4-point test of rectangular specimen

$\sigma = 2Pa / (\pi r^3)$ in 4-point test of round specimen

where P = bending load at breaking (rupturing) point, L = distance between the supporting points, b = breadth of the rectangular bar sample, d = depth (height) of the rectangular bar sample, r = radius of cylindrical rod sample, and a = (distance between the supporting points − distance between the loading points).

3.4 THERMAL PROPERTIES

"Thermal property" is a general term used for a class of property where the response of a material to the application of heat is measured. When a material is placed at a higher temperature, it absorbs energy in the form of heat, its temperature rises, its dimensions increase, and the heat energy will be transferred from the hotter region to the cooler region of the specimen (if a temperature gradient exists), and ultimately the specimen may melt.

A refractory technologist must have the idea about the thermal properties of different refractory materials for selecting them in different applications; as application temperature is high, temperatures may fluctuate, and thermal gradients may prevail, which requires designing of the refractory lining. For the refractory, the commonly measured thermal properties are thermal expansion and thermal conductivity.

3.4.1 Thermal Expansion

Whenever a material is heated, it absorbs heat energy and the energy level (potential energy) of matter increases. This heat or thermal energy is consumed by the increased vibrational movements of the atoms. That means thermal energy is converted to the vibrational energy (potential energy, PE) of atoms. This increase in vibrational energy increases the amplitude of atomic vibration of each atom of the material about their mean position. Figure 3.3 shows the plot of potential energy against the interatomic distance of any material with varying temperature. The distance between two atoms varies during vibration and the minimum and maximum distances can be marked from the potential energy plot. Due to the asymmetric nature of this plot, the mean distance between the atoms increases with temperature from its most stable condition, and material expands on heating.

Say, for a material, the equilibrium distance of separation between its atoms (bond length) is r_0 at temperature $T = 0$ K. As the temperature is increased (as marked by T_1, T_2, T_3, T_4, and T_5), the atoms absorb available thermal energy, and therefore the potential energy of the material is also increased (say corresponding PE levels are E_1, E_2, E_3, E_4, and E_5) and the vibration of atoms will also be increased to higher energy levels. Atoms vibrate between two extreme positions marked by the PE curve corresponding to each energy level (Figure 3.3a). At temperature T_1, the atoms will vibrate between a_1 and b_1 positions, and at temperature T_2, they will vibrate between a_2 and b_2 positions, and so on. Now as the PE curve is asymmetric, the mean positions between a_1 and b_1, a_2 and b_2, and so on (at higher energy levels) shift to the right compared to that of equilibrium

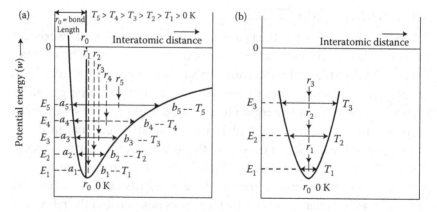

FIGURE 3.3 (a) PE plot and mean spacing between atoms for any material with increasing temperature. (b) PE plot of a strongly bonded material.

distance r_0. That is, the separation distance between the atoms increase with increasing temperature ($r_5 > r_4 > r_3 > r_2 > r_1$ at $T_5 > T_4 > T_3 > T_2 > T_1$). Thus, the dimension of the material increases with increasing temperature. Again, the stronger the atomic bond energy, the deeper and narrower will be the potential energy plot, and the lesser will be the asymmetry of the plot (Figure 3.3b). Hence, lesser will be the increase in the mean distance between the atoms on increasing temperature and lesser will be the thermal expansion values. So for refractories and ceramics, which are having stronger bonds (ionic or covalent bonds) than that of metals (metallic bonds), have lower thermal expansion values than metals.

Thermal expansion is commonly expressed as

$$\text{Percent linear thermal expansion} = (L_f - L_i) \times 100 / L_i,$$

and

$$\text{Coefficient of linear thermal expansion} = (L_f - L_i) / (L_i \cdot \Delta T),$$

where L_i = initial length of the sample, L_f = final length after reaching the maximum temperature, and ΔT = temperature difference.

The magnitude of the coefficient of thermal expansion remains constant for any specific material in a specific temperature range but increases with rising temperature. At lower temperatures, this increase is due to the higher amplitude of vibration of atoms at a higher energy level (temperature). For higher temperatures, the increased asymmetry in the PE curve is due to the increased amplitude of vibrations along with the formation of defects (Frenkel and Schottky) at higher temperatures, resulting in increased values of coefficient of thermal expansion. Again for samples containing non-isometric crystals, thermal expansion values vary with the crystallographic axis. The close-packed direction (higher bond strength) has a lower value of thermal expansion and this variation in the expansion values reduces with increasing temperature. The coefficient of thermal expansion values of some common refractory materials are given in Table 3.2. Also linear thermal expansion of different refractory materials is shown in Figure 3.4.

3.4.2 Thermal Conductivity

Thermal conductivity is an intrinsic property of a material and related to the transfer of heat. Heat flows from a higher side to a lower side, and the

TABLE 3.2 Coefficient of Linear Thermal Expansion
Values of Some Common Refractories

Name	Coefficient of Linear Thermal Expansion (α), $°C^{-1} \times 10^{-6}$
Alumina (corundum), Al_2O_3	8.8
Fused silica	0.4
Magnesia, MgO	13.5
Zirconia, ZrO_2 (stabilized)	11
Mullite, $3Al_2O_3 \, 2SiO_2$	5.3
Spinel, $MgO \, Al_2O_3$	7.6
Silicon carbide, SiC	5.12

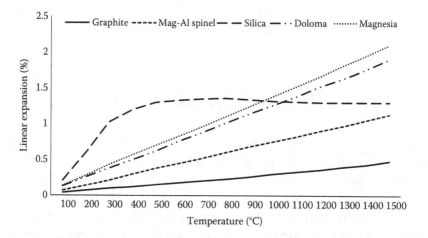

FIGURE 3.4 Linear thermal expansion of different refractory materials against temperature.

material that carries the heat is called a conductor. Thermal conductivity is the measure of the ability of a material to carry the heat from its hotter side to the cooler side. Heat conduction takes place when a temperature gradient exists between two opposite surfaces of a solid (or stationary fluid) medium. Conductive heat flows from a high-temperature to a low-temperature region as the higher temperature is associated with higher energy level or greater molecular movement. Energy is transferred from the more energetic molecules to the less energetic ones when neighboring molecules collide or come into contact with each other. Thermal conductivity is described as the amount of heat energy transferred per unit time per unit surface area at a unit distance between the surfaces with a unit difference of temperature.

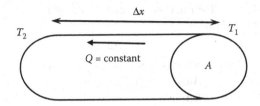

FIGURE 3.5   Sketch of heat flow (thermal conduction) through a material.

Thermal conductivity (K, unit W/[m.K]) describes the transport of heat energy through a body per unit time per unit area under a unit temperature gradient, as shown in Figure 3.5. It is expressed as the amount of heat (Q) transported (flowing perpendicularly at a steady rate) per unit of time (t) [that is dQ/dt or heat flow] through an unit area (A) of cross section [so $dQ/A\ dt$, that is, heat flux] at an unit temperature gradient ($\Delta T/\Delta x$, where ΔT is the temperature difference between two surfaces [$T_1 - T_2$] and Δx is the distance between two surfaces). So thermal conductivity,

$$K = \frac{\left(\dfrac{dQ}{dt}\right)}{A\left(\dfrac{\Delta T}{\Delta x}\right)}$$

Based on thermal conductivity values materials are classified into two major groups. Materials having high thermal conductivity are called conductors and are used mainly to transfer heat from one side to the other and also act as a heat sink. The other type of material having very low thermal conductivity values are called insulators, which are used for thermal protection, that is, to prevent any heat loss from any system (best examples are refractories). The approximate values of thermal conductivity of some common materials are given in Table 3.3. Also, the variation of thermal conductivity of different refractory materials against temperature is shown in Figure 3.6.

3.5 THERMOMECHANICAL PROPERTIES

The most significant properties of refractories are those that allow them to work in the application environments at elevated temperatures. Among them withstanding mechanical load at high temperature is most important. Refractories must have sufficient strength to withstand the load of the furnace and also the mechanical action of the charge and process

TABLE 3.3 Thermal Conductivity Values for Some
Common Materials

	Graphene
1000	Silver, copper, gold, silicon carbide
	Aluminum, graphite
100	Silicon
	Metals, iron
	Steel, carbon bricks
10	Silicon nitride
	Aluminosilicates
	Refractories
1.0	Ice, glass, fire clay, concrete
	Water
	Polymer, coal, brick, epoxy
0.1	Polyethylene, building boards, oils, wood
	Fiber boards, insulations
	Air, polystyrene, organic foam, paper, cotton
0.01	Krypton, freon (gaseous)
0.001	Vacuum insulation

Thermal conductivity at RT (W/mK) (vertical axis label)

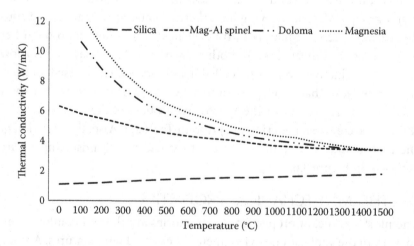

FIGURE 3.6 Variation of thermal conductivity of different refractory oxides
against temperature.

materials at the processing conditions. Hence, evaluation of mechanical properties at the application temperatures is a critical parameter for selecting the refractory.

Refractories are made from natural materials and the presence of impurities, even in a minute amount, is very common. Though the raw materials for a specific refractory are very pure, even a minute amount of impurity is sufficient in forming a little amount of low melting phase in the refractory. This may cause deformation of shape and degradation in the strength of the refractory at elevated temperatures. Both of these will result in sagging or collapse of the refractory structure. Hence, measurement of strength at high temperatures gives the idea of the safe highest application temperature of a refractory. There are two common techniques for measuring strength at high temperatures. These are the hot modulus of rupture and compressive creep.

3.5.1 Hot Modulus of Rupture (HMOR)

This is nothing but the measurement of modulus of rupture, as described in cold MOR (Section 3.3.2) in the hot condition. The whole testing is done in a furnace at the desired test temperature. Three-point bending test is done on a rectangular bar samples for HMOR. This measurement is important as it also incorporates the tensile condition of the refractory sample along with the compressive one, which is not included in other hot strength measurements. Specially designed furnaces, named HMOR furnace, are used for this testing having sample support and loading rods inside the furnace made of high-temperature ceramic materials. The formula and calculation used for such measurements are the same as that of the cold MOR.

3.5.2 Creep

The common feature of the application conditions of different refractories is high temperature and load. This condition continues for a long time, and in some cases, for years together. Hence occurrence of any deformation under heat and load for prolonged period is important for understanding the structural integrity of the refractory lining. Creep is the measurement of the deformation of any material against time under a specific load and temperature conditions. Hence, for refractories creep is one of the ideal characterization techniques to evaluate its performance. The creep measurement is little different for refractories than that of the metals, as for refractories, it is conventionally compressive creep, but for metals, it is generally in the tensile mode.

When a material is placed under a load of fixed stress value at a temperature above $0.4T_m$ (where T_m is the melting point of the material in Kelvin scale), the strain of the material continues to increase with increasing time at a rate depending on the inherent characteristics of the material. This slow and continuous deformation of a material against time under constant load and heat is defined as a creep. Creep is an inelastic property of a material and sometimes also expressed as viscoplasticity of a material. This is because when a material deforms under heat and load, it behaves like a plastic material (viscous flow), and the deformation is permanent in nature (not an elastic one). This deformation is due to the presence of liquid phase in the material at high temperature under load due to which grains slide and deform. Again deformation occurs due to the reduction in viscosity of the liquid under load at high temperatures. A refractory material has better creep resistance even on a higher amount of liquid phase formation if the liquid has a higher viscosity (resulting in lower flowability and deformation). So the amount and viscosity of the liquid phase present (which depends on the type and amount of the impurity phases) control the deformation and creep behavior of the refractory materials to a great extent.

3.6 ABRASION PROPERTIES

Abrasion is the damage or destruction of a material due to friction during use. It is related to the interactions between surfaces and is caused due to the deformation and removal of material from the surface as a result of the mechanical action of the opposite surfaces. The relative motion between the two surfaces and initial mechanical contact between them are important. Abrasion wear can also be defined as a process where the interaction between two surfaces or bounding faces of solids within the working environment results in dimensional loss of one solid, with or without any actual decoupling and loss of material. Abrasion is dependent on the working environment present, like the direction of sliding, nature of load (reciprocating, rolling, and impact), speed, and temperature, among others. Also different types of counterbodies such as solid, liquid, or gas and type of contact ranging between single phase and or multiphase are important.

Refractories face continuous friction due to the movement of the charge or product materials during use and also under the mechanical thrust of the processing conditions at high temperatures. The rubbing action of the charge and product particles on the porous surfaces of the refractory material causes the removal of material and wear. Descending solid charge materials in a blast furnace is a common example for sliding abrasion and wear of refractory.

Also, refractories encounter impact wear, which is, in reality, a short sliding motion where two surfaces interact at an exceptionally short time interval but with a higher mechanical thrust. Wear increases with sliding distance between the surfaces, load, and is inversely proportional to the strength, densification, and hardness of the refractory. Wear is defined as the loss of substance from surfaces in contact with relative motion. When two different surfaces, one hard and another soft, are in contact and in relative motion, the softer asperities undergo fracture or deformation and wear. Dense, high strength, fine-grained, and high hardness refractories show better wear resistances. Loss of refractory material due to mechanical action (wear), measured in weight, compared with density value and finally expressed as volume loss, is defined as the abrasion loss of refractory.

3.7 CORROSION PROPERTIES

The corrosion behavior of any refractory is important for the performance and life in any application area. Corrosion behavior is the chemical property of any refractory dependent on the chemical affinity (character), densification behavior, pore character (amount, size, and distribution of the pores), impurities amount and types, strength behavior, etc. and cannot be determined just by viewing or touching the substance. As it affects the internal structure of any material (unlike the physical properties) and may affect all other properties, a detailed understanding and evaluation of corrosion behavior of a refractory is required.

Refractories are used for any high-temperature processing where they face different chemical environments and are in contact with chemically active solids, liquids, or gases. Hence for refractories, resistance to these chemicals are very important for their structural integrity, performance, and life of the whole refractory and furnace structure. Refractories need to have chemical corrosion resistances that are prevalent in any specific application. A chemical reaction with the solid, liquid, or gaseous environments may result in new phases in the refractory, volumetric instability due to change in volume, the formation of the liquid phase, deformation, and obvious degradation of properties. A direct reaction between solid materials with refractories are less probable, but corrosion due to gases and liquids is prominent and important for the performance and life of the refractory. There are different techniques available for characterizing the corrosion resistance of a refractory material. As per the application environments, refractories used for stack area of a blast furnace (gaseous attack from carbon monoxide) and any slag or glass (liquid phase) contact areas are most important for the evaluation of chemical resistances.

3.7.1 Carbon Monoxide (CO) Disintegration

The best example of corrosion of refractory by the gaseous material is the upper stack area of blast furnace where the refractories are attacked by carbon monoxide (CO) gas, present in that region (CO is generated from the carbothermal reduction reaction of iron-making process in a blast furnace). The degradation in quality and disintegration of the refractory by CO is mainly dependent on the amount of ferric oxide present in the refractory.

The maximum temperature in the upper stack area of blast furnace reaches up to around 600°C, and fire clay-based refractories are most suitable for such low-temperature applications from the property requirements and economic points of view. The sources of fire clay are generally contaminated with good amount of iron oxide, and this iron oxide reacts with CO present in the environment at the temperature range of 450–550°C to form iron carbide (cementite) phase. This reaction is associated with volumetric expansion, which causes cracking and disintegration of the refractory.

$$6Fe_2O_3 + 4CO = 4Fe_3C + 11O_2$$

Even though there is no disintegration of the refractory, there may be discoloration or carbon deposition in it, which drastically deteriorates the properties. So fireclay refractories with a limited amount of iron oxide are to be selected for such applications.

3.7.2 Slag or Glass Corrosion

In many of the high-temperature applications, refractories are in contact with liquid phases and in mostly with corrosive liquids. Very common examples are slag (which is mainly basic in nature for iron and steel industries), glass (which is acidic in nature), etc. These chemically active liquids at high temperatures reacting with the refractory materials cause corrosion and they penetrate within the refractory through the pores and corroded structure, resulting in drastic deterioration of the properties. Hence, it is important for any refractory manufacturer and user to know how much the corrosive liquid can penetrate, react, or corrode and degrade the refractory.

Any liquid can penetrate a refractory if the liquid is highly fluid and there are openings (like pore or cracks) on the refractory surfaces. Hence, penetration of liquid slag or glass is dependent on the amount and size of surface pores (apparent porosity) present and presence and size of any crack. The corrosive liquid can only penetrate through a pore or crack if the size of the pore or crack is larger than that of the minimum droplet size of the slag or glass at that temperature (consideration of surface energies). The higher the temperature, lower is the viscosity of the liquid and lower will be a minimum size of the droplet, so higher is the (chance of) penetration. Slag or glass penetrated refractory portion will have a different character than that of the rest of the unaffected refractory that causes cracking, disintegration, and degradation of the whole refractory structure.

Again refractories, as a whole or any component of it, may react with the corrosive liquid (slag or glass) and may get dissolved or washed (eaten) away. Impurities present in the refractories are prone to be attacked by the corrosive liquids and degrades the quality of the refractory faster. Corrosion reaction may proceed through the matrix phase or grain boundaries of the refractory microstructure, where the concentration of the impurities is high though the main granular phase may remain unaffected and unaltered. Microstructural studies can confirm exactly which component of corrosive liquid is more penetrating or more corrosive to the refractory or which types of impurity phases are affected most and what kind of reactions are occurring within the refractory microstructure due to the presence of the corrosive liquid or its components. For the case of alumina refractory being corroded by steel making slag, if lime-bearing aluminosilicates are found in the refractory corroded portion, then lime and silica are the components of slag that cause the degradation most. Again the formation of calcium hexa-aluminates in the structure, if found in microstructure/phase analysis study, is beneficial to restrict the progress of the penetrating slag and its components due to the volume expansion during the formation, filling the pores and voids, and limits the ingress of slag in the refractory.

3.8 REFRACTORY-SPECIFIC PROPERTIES

Till now the properties described are common to other materials also, and they are studied in certain other fields too. But there are some properties commonly and specifically used and measured for the refractory materials only. These refractory-specific properties are not required, useful, and measured for any other types of materials. These properties, which are described below, are very common and conventional to refractories and are used in any specification of the refractories.

3.8.1 Refractoriness or Pyrometric Cone Equivalence

This is the inherent property of any material by which it can withstand high temperature having no appreciable deformation or softening without any external load. Refractoriness is also called softening temperature or pyrometric cone equivalent (PCE) temperature and is measured as a specific temperature that indicates the starting of fusability of any refractory material without any external load. In other words, it is the temperature when a material starts to soften under the action of heat under only its own weight. For a very pure material, the refractoriness matches (very close) with the fusion (melting) temperature. Hence, this property may also come under the broad category of thermal properties of refractories. Table 3.4 shows the melting (fusion) temperature of some commonly used refractory materials.

Refractories are made from natural materials and are commonly associated with impurities. Even in the case of synthetic materials, purity level is significantly high, but the material is not completely free from impurities. So refractories are always associated with some impurities. The presence of an impurity or a secondary material generally lowers the fusion temperature, as commonly found in phase diagrams. Hence, the refractories used commercially (having impurities in them) do not have any sharp melting temperature and start to soften at a lower temperature (melt progressively over a range of temperature) than that of the pure material's

TABLE 3.4   Melting Point Values of Some Pure Refractory Materials

Name	Melting Point (°C)
Alumina (corundum), Al_2O_3	2050
Silica, SiO_2	1713
Magnesia, MgO	2825
Zirconia, ZrO_2	2550
Chrome oxide, Cr_2O_3	2427
Lime, CaO	2570
Mullite, $3Al_2O_3 \cdot 2SiO_2$	1810
Spinel, MgO Al_2O_3	2135

melting point. The effect of the impurity or a secondary material on the softening of refractory materials depends on the following factors,

1. Chemical nature of the impurity phase (strong reduction in softening point occurs when impurities are in opposite chemical nature to that of the main constituent, say a basic impurity in an acidic refractory and vice versa)

2. Amount of the impurity present

3. Fusion point of the lowest fusing constituents present in the system

4. The capacity of the lowest fusing constituent to react and dissolve the higher fusing components

Refractoriness is measured by comparing the softening character of an unknown material against some known materials, making the samples in pyramid cone shapes. These pyramid-shaped cones are termed as pyrometric cones. The characterization is involved in comparing the softening behavior of the test material cones against standard reference cones, searching for the equivalency between standard and unknown cones, so this property is termed as pyrometric cone equivalent (PCE). This pyrometric cones were first developed by Herman August Seger and accordingly the standard cones are named as Segar cones. Also, there are Orton cones, which are globally accepted and used. Each standard cone has a number that corresponds to a specific temperature where that specific numbered cone will soften. This is done by very careful and precise selection of highly pure raw materials and mixing them in such a proportion that the particular numbered cone will soften on that specific temperature only. The softening temperature of a specific cone number may vary for different standard cone systems as they are manufactured with different compositions and from different sources of raw materials.

The pyrometric cones have a triangular base and a defined dimension and size. On heating, the cones that are placed at a little inclination (not vertical) will bend due to softening at high temperatures. This bending and lowering of the tip of the pyramid shaped cones will continue on increasing the temperature. Now, the tip of a specific cone will touch the base at a specific temperature. Every cone number of any standard cone system has a fixed tip-touching temperature (at which the tip touches the base). Any test (unknown) sample's cone, when matches with a standard cone in tip-touching temperature, is considered to have the refractoriness equivalent to that of the standard cone number (or its temperature). When the refractoriness (tip-touching temperature) of the unknown sample falls in between two standard cone numbers, it is expressed as in-between those two standard cone numbers (associated temperatures).

Cone manufacturers follow strictly the standard procedures to control variability (within the same batch and between batches) and to ensure that cones of a given grade remain consistent in their properties over long periods. Even though cones from different manufacturers can have relatively similar numbering systems, they are not identical in their softening characteristics. If a change in the cone system is done from one manufacturer to another, then the differences in tip-touching temperatures must be considered. Table 3.5 shows the cone numbers and their corresponding temperatures of commonly used standard cone systems.

Though this property gives an idea about the maximum allowable temperature limit of a refractory (without any external load) but in a practical sense, this temperature has little relevance. There is no such application where a refractory is used without any external load. Hence this measurement, though gives an idea about the inherent characteristic of a particular refractory system, is not very useful for practical applications.

3.8.2 Refractoriness under Load

Refractoriness under load (RUL) is an important property of a refractory from the practical application point of view. This property measures the refractoriness under a specific load, as the name suggests. In this method, initiation (measured as temperature) of deformation or softening of a refractory composition is evaluated under a constant load against an increasing temperature. As both temperature and load are involved in RUL, it may come under the broad category of thermomechanical properties. RUL indicates the safe temperature of use for a refractory under the combined effect of heat and a fixed load. The specific load maintained for RUL is 0.2 MPa.

In practical applications, refractories are always under some load, from the dead weight of the furnace and refractory lining, from the charge and product materials, from the air, flame, flue gas pressure, etc. Moreover, this load is unevenly distributed through the refractory lining and changes with time; sometimes cyclic loading is also present (say, for rotary kilns, steel ladles, etc.). Grains within the refractory will slide over one another under the application of external load whenever a minute amount liquid phase is present in-between them (low melting compounds

TABLE 3.5　End Point of PCE Measurement for Different Cone Systems Used in Refractories

Cone No.	End Point (°C)			
	Orton (US)	Segar (Germany)	British	French
12	1337	1375		
13	1349	1395		
14	1398	1410		
15	1430	1440		
16	1491	1470		
17	1512	1500		
18	1522	1520		
19	1541	1540		
20	1564	1560	1530	1530
23	1605	–		1580
26	1621	1580	1580	1595
27	1640	1600	1610	1605
27½	–	1620		
28	1646	1640	1630	1615
29	1659	1660	1650	1640
30	1665	1680	1670	1650
31	1683	1700	1690	1680
31½	1699	–		
32	1717	1710	1710	1700
32½	1724	1720		
33	1743	1730	1730	1745
33½	–	1740		
34	1763	1760	1750	1760
35	1785	1780	1770	1785
36	1804	1800	1790	1810
37	1820	1830	1825	1820
38	1835	1860	1850	1835
39	1865	1880		
40	1885	1900		
41	1970	1940		
42	2015	1980		

due to the presence of impurities) at high temperatures. This will cause a deformation of the refractory and will limit the application of the refractory at further high temperatures. Again the viscosity of the liquid phase also plays a vital role on sliding of grains and deformation of refractory. The very minimum amount of impurity and high viscosity of the fused

TABLE 3.6   Refractoriness and RUL (T_a) Values of Some Common Refractories

Refractory/Major Constituent	Purity (%)	Refractoriness (°C)	RUL, (T_a) (°C)
Silica	SiO_2-94	1680	1650
	SiO_2-97	1710	1680
Fire clay	Al_2O_3-30	1680	1350
	Al_2O_3-40	1740	1450
	Al_2O_3-45	1760	1480
High alumina	Al_2O_3-50	1760	1500
	Al_2O_3-60	1785	1420
	Al_2O_3-70	1804	1550
	Al_2O_3-80	1820	1550
	Al_2O_3-85	1820	1580
	Al_2O_3-90	>1850	1700
	Al_2O_3-95	>1850	1720
MgO	90	>1850	1600
	95	>1850	1650
	97	>1850	1680
MgO–Cr_2O_3	MgO-60 (min) Cr_2O_3-15 (min)	>1850	1700
	MgO-50 (min) Cr_2O_3-6 (min)	>1850	1650
MgO–Cr_2O_3 (direct bonded)	MgO-60 (min) Cr_2O_3-20 (min)	>1850	1720
	MgO-72 (min) Cr_2O_3-11 (min)	>1850	1700
	MgO-55 (min) Cr_2O_3-24 (min)	>1850	1750

mass/liquid phase will result in excellent RUL values in the refractory. The measurement of deformation is calculated from the dimensional change of the refractory during heating under load and two different temperatures, named temperature of appearance (T_a) and temperature of the end (T_e), are specified as the initiation of deformation and end of deformation. T_a has greater importance as this can be taken as the highest safe temperature of application for any refractory. Refractoriness and RUL (T_a) values of some common refractories are shown in Table 3.6.

In general, refractories have a lower RUL value compared to its refractoriness (PCE value). Deformation due to sliding of grains under load at high temperatures on the formation of a liquid phase in the refractory matrix is responsible for such a wide difference. Refractories deform at a much faster rate, even in the presence of a very minute amount of liquid, when they are under mechanical load. Hence, RUL is a much better parameter to judge a refractory than refractoriness. But still the measurement technique of RUL is far from the actual service conditions. In application, the load on refractories is not constant for its life. It may also vary from one portion to another, and may also be cyclic in nature (say in rotary kilns). The whole refractory is not in a temperature equilibrium condition, with only one surface getting heated and a major portion of the load is carried by the relatively cooler portion of the refractory. So RUL, though better than refractoriness, gives only an indication of the temperature at which the bricks will start to deform in service conditions with similar kind of a fixed load. It gives only a comparative index of quality among different refractories. Also, RUL does not consider any time factor, which is equally important at that high temperature. The use of refractory for a prolonged time is the general requirement and deformation starts at a much lower temperature on prolonged use, due to fatigue. So judging of the actual performance of a refractory is difficult to understand from the RUL value. In this regard, creep (discussed in Section 3.5.2) is better, as it incorporates time factor in the measurement of deformation at high temperature under load.

3.8.3 Thermal Shock Resistance

This property can also be called as thermal spalling resistance or thermal fatigue resistance. Degradation in the quality of a refractory due to repeated (cyclic) change in thermal state is measured by this property. During the use of refractories, heating and cooling cycles occur, along with a rapid change in temperature, which causes uneven expansion and contraction of the refractory, resulting in a huge thermal stress and associated strain and finally cracking, fracturing, and breaking of the refractory. This strain may be more critical if the refractory composition is not uniform and there is a phase transformation in the refractory composition within the temperature range of thermal cycle, which cause non-uniformity in its thermal expansion character. This non-uniform expansion behavior may result in cracks and failure of the refractory.

Thermal spalling is dependent on the environmental conditions in which thermal cycles are occurring, like the temperature difference between hot and cool conditions, heating and cooling rate of thermal cycles, the medium of thermal cycle conditions (like water and air), etc. Thermal spalling is dependent on the following refractory properties.

1. Thermal expansion: The higher the thermal expansion characteristics higher will be the dimensional change on change in temperature. Now if the temperature drop is very fast, then the refractory will have nearly no time to adjust to the dimensional change and will have a tremendous strain within it. This strain will keep on

multiplying as the number of the thermal cycles will progress and will finally result in cracking, breaking, or bursting of the refractory. Hence to have a better thermal shock resistance, the refractory should have low thermal expansion characteristics.

2. Thermal conductivity: In thermal cycles, the surface of the refractory will reach the outside temperature instantly but the interior will change slowly and will remain in the previous conditions for a prolonged period. This difference in thermal state between the interior and the exterior of a refractory will cause strain and may lead to failure. Now if the thermal conductivity of the refractory is high, the interior of the refractory will also reach the ambient thermal conditions very fast, resulting in a very minimum strain, reduced cracking, and reduced chances of failure. Hence for better thermal shock resistance, a refractory must have high thermal conductivity values.

3. Strength: If the refractory has higher mechanical strength characteristics, the crack that may be generated by the thermal spalling will be resisted and restricted to progress through the refractory and failure will be delayed. Hence, a strong refractory will fail at a higher strained conditions and will result in better thermal shock resistance.

4. Elastic modulus: During thermal cycles, the refractory will be prone to change its dimension as per the ambient or outside thermal conditions. Now if a refractory has a high value of elastic modulus, then the requirement for sudden and repeated dimensional changes caused by the thermal conditions of each cycle will be less accommodated by the refractory, resulting in cracking and failure of the refractory.

5. Porosity: For any dense refractory, the presence of porosity helps in increasing thermal shock resistance. Closed pores that are present in the interior of the refractory actually act as a crack arrestor or stress absorber by blunting the crack (generated by thermal shock) tip during its progress through the refractory. The sharp tip of the crack, when interacting with the closed pores, becomes blunt and directionless and requires much higher level of strain energy to propagate further. Again any crack that is getting generated from the surface of a refractory will have less energy to form if the refractory has higher apparent (surface) porosity. As the strain energy available from the strain of thermal shock to initiate the crack will be

distributed amongst the surface pores (who act as a crack generator) and energy available for each pore to generate the crack will be less. Thus, a higher level of total strain energy will be required to initiate the crack, resulting in much higher thermal shock resistance. Also, porosity can absorb the expansion in volume due to increase in temperature, causing a reduction in thermal strain and an increase in thermal shock resistances.

For insulating refractories, the porosity level is quiet high, which results in the poor strength of the refractories. Hence, higher porosity in insulating (non-dense) refractory is actually of no benefit and increase in porosity in a porous body will further deteriorate the strength properties.

The thermal strain may also be generated in a refractory sample if a huge temperature gradient exists between its two surfaces. The dimension of the hot face will be higher than that of the cold one (wide difference in dimensions if the thermal expansion coefficient is high) and temperature difference between the surfaces will be higher when the thermal conductivity is low for the material. Thus the strain generated will be enormous. Again this strain will keep on increasing with the increase in cyclic temperature change or prolonged use, resulting in failure of the material.

3.8.4 Permanent Linear Change on Reheating

This is a typical property especially required for the refractories. It can be visualized as the dimensional change (in general shrinkage) of the refractory on second firing. Shrinkage (discussed in Section 3.2.3) is the dimensional change of a refractory that occurs due to firing (from dried condition). As permanent linear change on reheating (PLCR) is the shrinkage value of the second firing, this property may be considered as the general category of physical properties. For the refractory manufacturing, it is important to obtain the desired dimensional size of the product. But for the user, it is important to know whether there will be any further (above acceptable limit) permanent dimension change of the refractory during its use. Any dimensional change, say shrinkage, at high temperature that may occur during use of the refractory will cause a gap between the refractories, resulting in heat leakage and many other associated problems. Again any expansion during application may cause instability and collapse of the refractory structure. During use, shrinkage may occur due to poor densification or sintering and expansion may be due to any incomplete reaction in the refractory composition, if those are not completed during firing of the manufacturing process.

Hence, if any fired refractory, ready for use at the application site, is again fired close to its application or firing temperature, it should have nearly no dimensional change. Any dimensional change that occurs due to this second firing (reheating) is termed as permanent linear change reheating (PLCR). If PLCR value is above the acceptable limit (which is very minimum), the refractory lot will be rejected. If the refractory manufacturer uses lower temperature of firing or lesser dwelling or soaking time during firing (to reduce the total firing cost) poor sintering or densification and incomplete reactions (if any) will occur, resulting in high PLCR values.

3.9 SUMMARY

Multiple application areas of refractory demand different kinds of properties. For dense refractories, the following properties are required.

- High bulk density (BD), low porosity (AP), low permeability, low shrinkage, and low specific gravity.

- Good mechanical properties like cold crushing strength (CCS) and cold modulus of rupture (CMOR).

- Low thermal expansion property is desired.

- High thermal conductivity for better thermal shock resistance or low thermal conductivity is required for better heat retention.

- High thermomechanical properties, like hot modulus of rupture (HMOR) and creep.

- High resistances against wear, abrasion, and chemical attack.

- High refractoriness (or PCE), refractoriness under load (RUL), thermal spalling (or shock) resistance, and low permanent linear change on reheating (PLCR).

Again for better performance in insulating refractory, it should have high AP, low thermal conductivity, high mechanical and thermomechanical properties, and other properties similar to dense refractories are desired (though for any refractory with high porosity the strength, hot strength, wear, chemical resistances, etc. are poor).

QUESTIONS AND ASSIGNMENTS

1. Why do we need different types of properties for refractories?

2. Briefly describe the properties required for dense refractories and insulating refractories.

3. Discuss the importance of thermal conductivity of refractories.

4. What the different physical properties and why they are important?

5. Why are thermomechanical properties more important for refractories than conventional mechanical properties?

6. Describe the requirements for resistance to chemical attack.

7. Why are wear properties required for refractories?

8. Discuss in detail the difference amongst HMOR, creep, and RUL. Discuss which property is more appropriate to importance and relevance of each of these properties.

9. What do you understand by thermal shock resistance? Describe the refractory properties on which thermal shock resistance is dependent and how?

10. What is PLCR? How is it different from shrinkage? Why is it important?

11. Why is carbon monoxide disintegration test important for fireclay refractories?

12. Why are the dimensions of the sample for measuring mechanical properties important?

BIBLIOGRAPHY

1. C. A. Schacht, *Refractories Handbook*, CRC Press, Boca Raton, FL, 2004.
2. J. H. Chesters, *Refractories—Production and Properties*, Woodhead Publishing Ltd., Cambridge, UK, 2006.
3. P. P. Budnikov, *The Technology of Ceramics and Refractories*, 4th edn., translated by E. Arnold, *Scripta Technica*, The MIT Press, Cambridge, MA, 2003.
4. *Harbison-Walker Handbook of Refractory Practice*, Harbison-Walker, PA, 2005.
5. S. C. Carniglia and G. L. Barna, *Handbook of Industrial Refractories Technology: Principles, Types, Properties, and Applications*, Noyes Publications, Saddle River, NJ, 1992.

6. A. Rashid Chesti, *Refractories: Manufacture, Properties and Applications*, Prentice-Hall of India, New Delhi, India, 1986.
7. W. David Kingery, H. K. Bowen, and Donald R. Uhlmann, *Introduction to Ceramics*, 2nd edn., John Wiley & Sons Inc., New York, 1976.
8. F. Singer and S. S. Singer, *Industrial Ceramics*, Springer, Berlin, 1963.
9. F. H. Norton, *Refractories*, 4th edn., McGraw-Hill, New York, 1968.

CHAPTER 4

Standards and Testing

4.1 INTRODUCTION TO DIFFERENT STANDARDS

Refractories are industrial materials used in high-temperature processing where the selection of a proper refractory is important for a particular application. This selection is done as per suitability of the refractory for that application, which can meet all the required property criteria of the application environment with the economy. Each application area demands a specific set of properties, which may be unique to that application only.

Most of the properties of a refractory are quantitative in nature (other than some visually descriptive ones like color, appearance, etc.). They are used as a metric by which the benefits of one type are measured and assessed by another type, and proper refractory selection is done for a particular application. The properties are a function of independent variables, like temperature, and often vary with the direction of the measurement and with the testing environment. Some of the properties are also dependent on the sample size.

Refractories are classic examples of ceramics that contain preexisting pores, flaws, and cracks in them arising from processing and manufacturing techniques. These deformities are not uniform among the batches of the same composition and even among the samples of the same batch. So the properties of each testing of the same sample may vary, and an average of few samples is a must to get accuracy and dependability in the results obtained.

Again, for an application, not a single property is important, rather a set of properties are required to be measured, and the measurement techniques must be acceptable to all, with accuracy and repeatability. So every measurement in each testing environment has to be done in precise and predetermined fixed conditions, which results in exactly similar values during each time of testing. So a set of fixed parameters is required for carrying out any testing, which will become like the "standards" for that testing.

A "standard" is a document that provides requirements, specifications, guidelines, or characteristics that can be used consistently to ensure that materials, products, processes, and services are fit for their purpose. It details the conditions and parameters for any testing, represents an indispensable level of information in that specific area, established by consensus mainly of the manufacturer, user, researchers, government agencies, and consumers. It is also certified and accepted by a recognized (government) organization that provides rules and guidelines for common and repeated use. Any standard is a collective work of different forum of people to meet the demands of the society and technology for better living.

The use of standards is becoming a prerequisite for trade, especially in the case of global business. A very large percentage of export is influenced by the international standards business. Above all, everyone can benefit from the conformity and integrity that standards will bring out. Use of standards helps our daily lives in many ways, making life easier, safer, and healthier by identifying and classifying products conforming to particular requirements and warrants service performance in long run.

Most of the technologically advanced countries are having their own standards. Most common and globally accepted standards that are used for refractories are

- British Standards Institutions of UK, code "BS."

- American Standards for Testing Materials of US, code "ASTM."

- Conformite Europeene (European Conformity) of European Economic Area, code "CE."

- International Organization for Standardization (ISO) standards of various countries, code "ISO."

- Deutsches Institut für Normung (German Institute for Standardization) of Germany, code "DIN."

- Association Française de Normalisation of France, code "AFNOR."

- Japanese Industrial Standards of Japan, code "JIS."

- GB (Guobiao) Standards of China, code "GB."

- Bureau of Indian Standards of India, code "IS."

All the different standards have their own method of testing refractory materials, and in many cases, the parameters are the same. The refractory material must follow and satisfy the standard norms of a particular country or a global zone to do business in that area.

4.2 TESTING OF REFRACTORIES

In the previous chapter, we have seen various types of refractory properties and the different subclasses of each type to characterize a refractory material. Each of the classes and subclasses is important for different refractories from the application points of view. Evaluation of these different classes and subclasses of properties is done as per certain specific standards. There are different norms mentioned in the different testing standards that are used in different parts of the world. Here in the present chapter, the testing methods are described in a much generalized way mostly for the shaped and fired refractories, covering mainly the popular and most widely used properties and the standards. The most common properties that are important and used for refractories have been discussed in Chapter 3 and the testing methods to evaluate them are discussed in the following.

4.3 TESTING OF PHYSICAL PROPERTIES

4.3.1 Bulk Density, Apparent Porosity, Water Absorption, and Apparent Specific Gravity

These properties are very commonly used to describe and judge a fired shaped refractory, like brick. Also, they are used for comparing the same quality of refractory obtained from different source or supplier to judge the quality for selection purpose in a specific application. The methods used to measure them are primary standard methods, suitable for quality control, research and development activity, comparison and selection, and compliance with specifications. Common assumptions associated with the test methods are the following:

1. Specimens do not react with water (otherwise non-aqueous liquid is to be used).

2. Maximum extent of original surfaces of the fired shaped article are retained in the test samples.

3. Requirements regarding the size and configuration are met.

4. Samples are not very fragile or having loose grains that may fall apart.

5. Surface pores are fully impregnated by boiling or vacuum method.

If any of the above stated assumptions are not fulfilled, the test results may be erroneous.

The presence of porosity in refractories does not allow us to measure the density and other related properties using simple Archimedes principle, as applied for non-porous samples. Hence, a modified Archimedes method is used for porous samples. The sample size required to measure these properties varies from one standard to another. Table 4.1 details the commonly used sample sizes mentioned in different popular standards. There are two main methods used for the determination of the above mentioned properties:

1. Boiling method

2. Vacuum or evacuation method

4.3.1.1 Boiling Method

The test specimen is cut from the main refractory retaining as much molded surfaces as possible. Then the sample is dried in an oven at 110°C and after reaching a constant mass, dried weight (D) is taken. The sample is then immersed completely in distilled water in the suspended condition such that none of the surfaces (even the bottom) touches the surface of the water container. The container is then heated, and the water is allowed to boil for 2 h. The sample should not touch the container walls also during the boiling period. If the water level goes down due to evaporation, the addition of water is to be done so that the samples must remain in the immersed condition all through the boiling period. After

TABLE 4.1 Sample Size for BD and AP Study as per Different Standard Specifications

Specification Standard	Sample Size
ASTM C 20–00 (reapproved 2015)	One quarter of a brick retaining four original surfaces
JIS 2205	One half or one quarter of a normal brick
IS 1528 part XV: 2007	65 mm × 65 mm × 40 mm

2 h of boiling, the container along with the suspended samples is allowed to cool down. After cooling, the suspended weight (S) of the sample is taken. This weight is taken while the sample remains in the suspended condition in water with the help of a loop or halter (made up of copper wire) hung from a balance. The balance must be counter-balanced with the wire in place and immersed in water to the same depth as is used when the test sample is in place.

Next the sample is taken out from water, and the extra surface water present is wiped off lightly from the surface by blotting with a wet or moistened towel, a smooth linen, or cotton cloth to remove all drops of water from the surface. Care must be taken such that blotting or wiping is only enough to remove the excess surface water that will drop from the surface. Excessive blotting or pressed wiping can produce an error by withdrawing water from the surface pores of the specimen. After wiping, the sample is again weighed for its soaked weight (W).

This W corresponds to the weight of the sample when the surface pores are filled with water. Hence, it is equal to the dry weight of the sample plus weight of water present in the surface pores. Now the term ($W - S$) indicates the mass difference of the sample measured in air and immersed in water when the surface pores are filled with water. Removal of air from the surface pores occurs during boiling as the volume of air present is increased due to heating and comes out of the surface as the sample is continuously heated during boiling, and air is replaced by water present nearby during the cooling period. Thus ($W - S$) indicates the bulk volume (without the volume of the surface pores) of the sample in CGS unit, as per Archimedes principle. Hence,

$$\text{Bulk density (BD)} = \left(\frac{\text{mass}}{\text{bulk volume}} \right) = \frac{D}{(W - S)}$$

Again the term ($W - D$) shows the weight of water present only in the surface pore of the sample. Hence, in CGS unit, the value of ($W - D$) is the volume of the water present in the surface pores, which is the volume of the total surface pores. Hence,

$$\text{Apparent porosity (AP) (\%)} = \frac{\text{volume of surface pores}}{\text{bulk volume}} = \frac{(W - D) \times 100}{(W - S)}$$

Water absorption (WA) is defined as the percentage of water absorbed by the sample per unit mass of it. So

$$WA = \frac{(W - D) \times 100}{D}$$

Apparent specific gravity (ASG) is defined as $D/(D - S)$

4.3.1.2 Vacuum/Evacuation Method

In this method, the measurement parameters and measuring conditions are exactly same as that of the boiling method. The only difference lies is the process part of the experiment. Here, the immersed samples are kept in vacuum instead of placing them for boiling immersed in water. Water or organic liquid (like kerosene, xylene) can be used as liquid for immersion of the test samples. Organic liquids cannot be used in boiling methods due to their high evaporation rate. For samples having hydration tendency or react with water, organic liquids have to be used instead of water and only vacuum method can be used for these measurements. Samples are immersed in liquid without touching the container surfaces (similar to boiling method) and the whole system is placed inside an empty vacuum desiccator, which is then evacuated to a vacuum level of 2.0 kPa (~25 mmHg column or 0.02 atmospheric pressure). This vacuum was maintained for at least 2 h, after which air is allowed to enter, and the measurements are done exactly in the similar way as mentioned in the boiling method. In this technique, the vacuum draws out the air from the surface pores and the void spaces are then filled with the surrounding liquid. If a liquid other than water is used, then the density of the liquid is required to be multiplied for the calculation of BD and ASG.

4.3.2 True Specific Gravity and True Density

True specific gravity (TSG) is the ratio of true density, determined at a specific temperature, to the density of water at that temperature and has no unit. It is a primary property related to chemical and mineralogical composition of the sample. Specific gravity helps to classify the refractories, can detect the differences in chemical composition and mineralogical phases or phase changes, and also is essentially required to calculate the total porosity and closed porosity of a refractory sample.

The test is done by immersing the powdered sample in a liquid, mostly water if the sample does not react with water. Few assumptions are also associated with the measurement process. The assumptions are (a) sample used is a true representative of a bulk material (only few grams are used), (b) nearly no porosity is present below the fineness of the powdered sample, (c) no impurity has been introduced during the preparation of the sample, etc. If the assumptions are not strictly valid, then the results may not be very accurate.

First, a representative piece of the refractory sample is to be taken. A higher number of samples may lead to better average value and accuracy in results. Each sample is to be crushed and ground first and then sieved through at least 150-micron sieve. No selective grinding and no exclusion of any portions, which may be difficult to crush or grind, is to be done. Particles passing through the sieve are demagnetized to remove any magnetic (iron) particles contaminated during crushing and grinding process. The powders are then collected and sampling is done to reduce the amount of sample for the test by coning and quartering method.

The sample (about 50 g) is dried at 110°C and then taken (poured) into a special glass bottle with a stopper rod, named pycnometer bottle [weight of the empty bottle W_1 (in g)], till the constant weight is achieved (W_2 in g). Next the bottle is filled with water (other liquid) in such a way so that the whole powder is immersed in liquid and the bottle is filled to half or two-thirds of its capacity. Then it is placed inside a vacuum desiccator and vacuum is started. Bubbles will start coming out from the sample through the liquid. A vacuum level of less than 25 m bar is maintained. With time, the removal of air bubbles will decrease and then it will die down. The vacuum is maintained for 1–2 h. The pycnometer bottle with the sample and liquid inside is shaken intermittently during the vacuum process to make sure that complete wetting of the material by the liquid has taken place. Instead of a vacuum, boiling can also be used, as used for BD and AP study, when water is used as the liquid medium.

Next, the pycnometer is taken out from the vacuum desiccator, and the sample particles are allowed to settle down if disturbed during vacuum or boiling process. Then the bottle is filled with the liquid, and the glass-stopper rod is placed. Care is necessarily required for filling and placing of glass-stopper so that there will not be any overflow of the sample powder out of the bottle and there is an overflow through the capillary tube when the stopper is inserted. The capillary of the stopper rod must be filled with the liquid. Any excess liquid coming out from the tip of the stopper rod or outside of the rod and outside of the bottle is wiped off with care so that it does not draw out any liquid from the capillary of the rod. Next the bottle with rod containing the sample and filled with liquid is weighed (W_3 in g). Then the pycnometer is emptied completely, washed, and dried. The clean and dried bottle is then filled with the test liquid, and the stopper rod is placed in such a way that the capillary inside the rod is filled as before. The weight of the filled pycnometer is taken (W_4 in g).

True specific gravity and true density are then calculated as per the following formula, and the results are reported to the nearest third decimal place:

$$\text{True specific gravity }(TSG) = \frac{(W_2 - W_1) \times D_1}{[(W_4 - W_1) - (W_3 - W_2)]}$$

and

$$\text{True density }(TD) = \frac{(W_2 - W_1)(D_1 - D_a)}{[(W_4 - W_1) - (W_3 - W_2)]} \text{ g/cm}^3$$

where, D_1 and D_a represent the densities of the liquid used and air respectively at the test temperature.

The ratio of bulk density to the true density represents the fraction of densification that has occurred in the sample. So the value $\{1 - BD/TD\}$ represents the fraction that has not densified or the fraction of total porosity present in the sample. Hence,

$$\text{Total porosity} = \left\{1 - \frac{BD}{TD}\right\} \times 100\%.$$

Now, this total porosity has two components. One is the surface or apparent porosity, for which the measurement process is described in Section 4.3.1. The other one is closed porosity, which remains within the sample and cannot be measured directly. Hence, this closed porosity can be calculated as total porosity—apparent porosity. So,

$$\text{Closed porosity} = \left[\left\{1 - \frac{BD}{TD}\right\} \times 100 - \text{apparent porosity}\right]\%$$

The sample preparation techniques used in this testing, that is crushing and grinding, only makes the sample finer than 150 microns, and the sample is not free from the closed pores that are finer than this size. The amount of residual closed pores may vary between the refractories and even within the samples of the same refractory. And the process mentioned above does not consider these fine pores. Hence, the values generated by the weights of different readings are close approximations rather than accurate representations of true specific gravity values. So for any comparison purposes and any refractory selection purposes, the results obtained by this method must be judiciously judged due to the presence of these fine closed pores and deviations from accuracy arising out of them should be kept in mind.

4.3.3 Permanent Linear Change on Reheating

Permanent linear change on reheating (PLCR) represents the permanent dimensional change of a fired refractory shape that may occur on second firing (reheating). Refractory shapes of different compositions exhibit unique permanent linear changes after reheating, which is primarily important for the refractory users. This test method provides a standard procedure for heating various classes of already fired refractories with appropriate heating schedules and measuring the dimensional changes. Dimensional changes may vary from batch to batch of the same source of material with the same composition of refractory due to processing inconsistency. And it is important to have an idea about the dimensional changes of the refractory during use.

Again the reheating is done with a specific heating schedule for a certain firing time, which may not be comparable to the actual application conditions. Also, the heating environment may vary from the actual applications. So the permanent change that may occur during application may differ from the testing results. But it helps to compare among different classes and subclasses of refractories and to select them for a specific application area. The measurement is essentially required for the refractory user industries and also for the developmental activities. The selection of representative sample for the test is important.

The different specifications have different dimensions for this test, as shown in Table 4.2, but all the specifications suggest to retain as many original or molded surfaces as possible. If the original refractory shape is smaller than the required dimensions, then the largest possible size is cut from that shape ensuring that the structure of the refractory is not damaged. Dimensions and volume of the samples are taken for the purposes of calculation. Then the samples are placed in the furnace in such a way that they are rested on the larger surface above a supporting brick (of the same refractory quality or, at least, similar refractoriness in quality). Furnace atmosphere needs to be oxidizing,

TABLE 4.2 Sample Size for PLCR as per Different Standard Specifications

Specification Standard	Sample Size
ASTM C 113–14 (reapproved 2014)	228 mm × 114 mm × 64 or 76 mm
JIS R 2208	114 mm × 20 mm × 20 mm
IS 1528 Part VI	50 mm × 50 mm × 125 mm

and the flame must not impinge on the sample surface. Non-reactive suitable refractory grains are placed in between the test samples and the supporting brick and also among the test samples. A specific gap (~40 mm) is also maintained between the samples. The furnace hearth should have a uniform temperature all-through, which is to be measured by a calibrated thermocouples or by a calibrated optical or radiation pyrometer. The final reheating temperature is dependent on the type of refractory that is being evaluated and its refractoriness. Every standard specification has some specific heating schedule, and the highest temperature of firing for this measurement for each type of refractory quality is about 50–100°C lower than the firing temperature of the refractory under testing. After the desired firing, the sample is allowed to cool down within the closed furnace and then it is taken out from the furnace. Any small blister formed on the surface of the samples is removed by rubbing with abrasive blocks, and the dimensions and volume are measured again. The PLCR is measured as

$$\frac{(L_f - L_i) \times 100}{L_i} \quad \text{for linear shrinkage}$$

and

$$\frac{(V_f - V_i) \times 100}{V_i} \quad \text{for volumetric shrinkage}$$

where L_f and V_f are the linear dimension and volume of the sample after reheating, and L_i and V_i are that of the before reheating firing.

4.4 TESTING OF MECHANICAL PROPERTIES

Mechanical properties are required to understand the strength of a material and essentially measured for the refractories in any applications. The two major ambient temperature strength measurement techniques are discussed here as detailed in the following.

4.4.1 Cold Crushing Strength

Cold crushing strength (CCS) values give an idea about of the suitability of a refractory for use in a specific application, only from the load-bearing capacity point of view. It is not a measure of performance at elevated temperatures. The results obtained from this testing must be judiciously used for comparison purpose as it depends on sample dimensions and shape, the nature of the testing surfaces (original fired, sawed, or ground), the orientation of the surfaces during testing, the loading pattern and rate, etc. Strength values may vary from source to source, batch to batch, and even within the same batch of a specific quality of refractory.

The test specimen size varies from one standard to another, and a few are mentioned in Table 4.3. Test samples of required size are cut from larger refractory shapes. If the original shape is smaller in dimension, the maximum size possible needs to be attained retaining the maximum number of original surfaces (molded and fired). In such cases, only one specimen shall be cut from a single fired shape without weakening or damaging the refractory. Test samples with cracks or other visible defects must be rejected for testing.

The sample must be completely dried and then cooled, and the surfaces of the sample that will receive the load from the testing machine shall be ground or cut to plane and parallel. If required, a sand-cement mortar or plaster of Paris paste is to be used to fill up any depression mark on the loading surface to make it perfectly flat. Asbestos fibreboards or cardboards 5 mm in thickness, and extending the sample size over the edges, are to be used as the bedding material at the bottom and top of the specimen. After placing the sample in the compression testing equipment with the bedding material, the load is applied (Figure 4.1). A spherical bearing block (lubricated for easy and accurate adjustment for proper placement) is to be used at the top of the test specimen in contact with the top surface and must be in the vertical axis of the test sample. The load is to be applied uniformly during the test. Loading is done to maintain a strain rate of 1.3 mm/min for both the dense and porous (insulating) refractories with a

TABLE 4.3 Sample Size for CCS as per Different Standard Specifications

Specification Standard	Sample Size
ASTM C 133-97 (reapproved 2015)	51 mm cube or cylinder with 51 mm dia. and height
JIS R 2206	60 mm cube
IS 1528 Part IV	230 mm standard brick or 75 mm cube

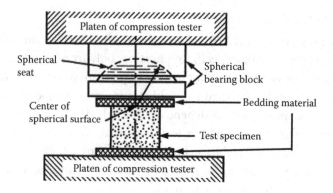

FIGURE 4.1   Testing arrangement for the measurement of CCS.

corresponding stress rate 12 MPa/min for dense and 3 MPa/min for insulating refractories. At a certain load, the sample will crush (break) or collapse and the maximum applied load value is noted. The CCS is reported as calculated by the following formula:

$$\text{Cold crushing strength} = \frac{W}{A}$$

where W = maximum load at the moment of crushing or breaking in kgf and A = average of the gross areas of top and bottom surfaces in m^2. The size of the test sample and the loading direction applied is to be mentioned in the test report.

4.4.2 Cold Modulus of Rupture

Cold modulus of rupture (MOR) test is performed on bar samples using a standard mechanical or hydraulic compression testing machine at a constant rate of stress increase. The maximum stress that a sample of specified dimensions can withstand is measured when it is bent in a three-point bending device until failure occurs. The method is used mainly for the shaped and fired refractories; for any chemically bonded or tar-bonded or unshaped products, a preliminary heat treatment may be required before testing.

The loading setup must have three bearing edges, two to support the test piece and one for the loading (Figure 4.2). The three edges have a specific radius of curvature as per the sample dimensions and have a length more than 5 mm greater than that of the breadth of the test sample. The contact

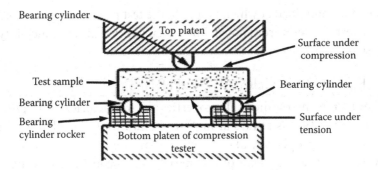

FIGURE 4.2   Testing arrangement for the measurement of cold MOR.

lines of the edges must be parallel to one other in a direction perpendicular to the length and the plane of the breadth of the test piece. The loading device must apply the load uniformly across the center of the sample and increase it at a uniform rate. The maximum load at the time of failure is recorded.

Each test piece shall be a whole standard rectangular brick [230 (228) mm × 114 mm × 76 mm or 230 (228) mm × 114 mm × 64 mm] or any one of the sizes 200 mm × 40 mm × 40 mm or 150 (152) mm × 25 mm × 25 mm. If test pieces are cut out from fired shapes, then the cutting must be done in such a way that the loading direction for testing must match with the pressing direction of the shape.

Test samples are first dried in an oven at 110°C and then cooled to avoid any moisture absorption. Next the breadth and height of each test piece are measured. Samples are then placed on the lower bearing edges of the loading equipment so that it rests symmetrically on two supporting (bearing) cylinders. When the test piece is a normal standard brick, the face bearing any brand mark, that is, the upper face, shall be in compression. If the test pieces have been cut out of the brick, the face of the test piece that corresponds to the original face of the brick (if it has been preserved) shall be in compression. Next the load is applied vertically to the test piece until failure occurs. The rate of increase load must conform to the following:

1. A stress rate of 9 MPa/min for a dense-shaped refractory (corresponding to a strain rate of 1.3 mm min) is maintained.

2. A stress rate of 3 MPa/min for a shaped insulating (porous) refractory (corresponding to a strain rate of 1.3 mm min) is maintained.

The maximum load at which failure of the test piece occurs is recorded and the test temperature is noted. The repeatability and reproducibility of the test are to be checked.

4.5 TESTING OF THERMAL PROPERTIES

The measurement of thermal properties for refractories is important as their application is always at high temperatures. Other than conventional thermal properties, like thermal expansion and thermal conductivity, refractoriness or PCE of a material is also considered as thermal properties.

4.5.1 Reversible Thermal Expansion

Reversible thermal expansion (RTE) is measured by dial gauge method using a horizontal type or vertical type dilatometer. A dilatometer is an equipment containing closed refractory tube at one end and refractory rod that holds and supports the test sample at the other, and the whole system is placed inside a furnace. For a temperature up to 1150°C, RTE is measured in a dilatometer with fused silica tube and fused silica rod that is connected to a dial gauge and the sample rests between the closed end of the fused silica tube and the fused silica rod. On an increase in temperature, any increase in the dimension of the sample will force the rod, and that will be indicated by the micrometer dial gauge, generally graduated in divisions of 0.01 mm. The temperature is measured by a thermocouple placed very close to that of the sample. When the temperature of thermal expansion measurement is higher than 1150°C, the vitreous silica system may crack due to the devitrifying effect within itself, so for temperatures above 1150°C high alumina system (mainly recrystallized alumina set ups) is used and horizontal dilatometer is used as well.

The test specimen (as a refractory cylinder) used has a dimension of 50 mm length and 10 mm diameter and is obtained from the refractory shape by core drilling or by cutting and grinding. The end faces of the sample must be very flat and parallel to each other.

The calibration of the apparatus is done before the experiment to check and measure any temperature variation between the outside of the refractory tube and the specimen and the expansion in length of the tube. A 50 mm standard piece (of fused silica or alumina as per the system) is used for calibration and any deviation from the zero reading on the dial gauge is noted against the temperature. The expansion values obtained in all subsequent tests with the apparatus shall be corrected by adjusting the difference between the dial gauge reading at a given temperature during the calibration test and the true expansion of 50 mm standard piece at that temperature.

For the test sample, the length is measured accurately by slide callipers and then is placed at the closed end of the tube in between the two refractory disks (to avoid any displacement during the test). Next refractory rod is placed at the free end of the disk on top of this specimen. A proper thermocouple is then inserted into the tube in such a way that the hot junction is positioned almost at the center of the specimen and is connected to a temperature recording device. Next the dial gauge is adjusted for zero reading. The whole system with the test sample is then placed in the furnace and heating is done at a predetermined rate (as per the specification), generally 5°C/min. The temperature and the corresponding dial gauge reading are noted at every 5 min.

The dial gauge reading is corrected according to calibration data, and the corrected values represent the linear dimensional change of the sample with the change in temperature. It is expressed as a percentage of the original length of the specimen. A graph relating to percent expansion value against temperature is also plotted for graphical representation.

4.5.2 Thermal Conductivity

The thermal conductivity of refractories is important as it determines the thermal transmission characteristics. This is important as the user industries select the refractories to attain a specified (precalculated) conditions of heat loss and corresponding cold face temperature, without exceeding the temperature limitation of the refractory used. So it is essential to know the heat conduction behavior of the refractory, heat loss, amount heat to be supplied to continue, and complete the high-temperature process. If a composite lining (multiple layers of refractory) is used, then the thermal conductivity of all the individual lining refractories is important to calculate the heat balance of the process. Different methods are used for measuring the thermal conductivity of refractories, as described in the following.

4.5.2.1 Calorimetric Method

This test method covers the determination of thermal conductivity of refractories under standardized conditions of testing using a calorimeter. It requires a large thermal gradient and steady state heat transmission conditions. The results are based on a mean temperature and are suitable for specification acceptance and selection of refractory type and design of multilayer refractory construction. The use of these data requires consideration of the actual application environment and the conditions.

A special apparatus is used for this method, having

1. An electrical heating chamber up to a maximum temperature of 1540°C in a neutral or oxidizing atmosphere and can maintain uniform heat distribution.

2. A copper calorimeter assembly that measures the amount of heat flowing through the test specimen by the water circulation process.

3. A water-circulating system with regulator valve to provide constant water supply to the calorimeter assembly at constant pressure and temperature conditions. The water is at ambient temperature with a minimum pressure of 30 kPa.

4. Calibrated thermocouples with hot junctions embedded in the test specimen and the cold junctions immersed in a mixture of ice and water.

5. A multiple differential thermocouples for measuring the temperature rise of the water flowing through the calorimeter.

Three numbers of standard bricks {230 (228) mm × 115 mm × 75 mm} and six numbers of soap bricks [230 (228) mm × 64 mm × 57 mm] with uniformity in structure and bulk density (measured after drying at 110°C), free of broken corners or edges, are used for the test. One straight brick is used as the test specimen, and one each of the other two bricks is used as guard brick on either side of the specimen. The six soap bricks are placed around the edges of the test specimen and guard bricks to prevent any side heat flow. The test specimen and guard bricks cover an area of approximately 456 mm by 342 mm.

The 230 (228) mm × 115 mm faces of the three straight bricks and the 230 (228) mm × 64 mm faces of the soap bricks are ground to flat and parallel. The sides that are to be placed in contact shall be ground flat and at right angles to the 230 (228) mm × 115 mm face of the straight brick and the 230 (228) mm × 64 mm face of the soap brick.

The following data are recorded for each 2-h test period (steady state of heat flow):

1. Linear dimensions of the test specimen

2. Distance between thermocouple junctions located in the test specimen

3. Three sets of temperature readings as measured by the thermocouples in the test specimen

4. Mean temperature between each pair of thermocouples in the test specimen as calculated from the temperatures recorded in (3)

5. Average rise in temperature of the water flowing through the calorimeter

6. Average rate of water flow through the calorimeter

7. The rate of heat flows through the test specimen per unit area

Thermal conductivity is calculated as

$$k = \frac{qL}{[A(t_1 - t_2)]}$$

where, k = thermal conductivity, W/m·K, q = rate of heat (W) flowing into the calorimeter (temperature rise in K of the water flowing through the calorimeter times the weight of flowing water kg/s), L = thickness (distance between hot junctions at which t_1 and t_2 are measured, in m), t_1 = higher of two temperatures measured in the test specimen (in K), t_2 = lower of two temperatures measured in the test specimen (in K), and A = area of center calorimeter (m²).

4.5.2.2 Parallel Hot Wire Method

It is a dynamic thermal conductivity measurement technique based on the measurement of the temperature increase at a certain location and a specified distance from a linear heat source embedded between two test pieces. The test pieces are heated in a furnace to the desired temperature and then local heating is done by passing electricity through a wire with known power embedded in the test piece along the length of the test piece. A thermocouple is fitted at a specified distance from the hot wire to measure the increase in temperature as a function of time, measured from the moment the heating current is switched on. From all these data, thermal conductivity is calculated.

The apparatus used for this technique consists of the following:

1. An electrically heated furnace that can heat the test assembly up to 1250°C.

2. A hot wire, platinum or platinum/rhodium, about 200 mm in length and max 0.5 mm in diameter. One end of the wire is attached to the lead for the supply of the heating current, and the other end is attached to a lead for measurement of voltage drop.

3. A stabilized AC power supply to provide current to the hot wire (preferably constant power supply).

4. Platinum/platinum–rhodium thermocouple (Type R or S), formed from a measurement thermocouple and a reference thermocouple connected in opposition.

5. A data acquisition system of temperature–time registration device with a sensitivity of at least 2 pV/cm and a temperature measurement to 0.05 K.

Each test assembly consists of two identical test pieces with standard brick dimensions or at least 200 mm × 100 mm × 50 mm in size. The surfaces of the test pieces, which are in contact with each other, must be very flat. A groove to accommodate the hot wire and the thermocouple shall be machined in both the contact faces.

The hot wire and differential thermocouple are placed between the two test pieces, with the hot wire along the center line of the brick faces in contact with each other. Next the test assembly is placed inside the furnace, resting each assembly on supports of the same material for uniform heating. Then the test assembly is connected to the measuring apparatus with the hot-wire circuit open. Next the furnace is heated to the test temperature at a maximum of 10 K/min.

After reaching the test temperature, a soaking of 10 min is done for uniformity of temperature. Then the heating circuit is closed, and a fixed power input (chosen as per recorder sensitivity) is provided in the hot wire circuit. The exact moment of initiation of the power supply is noted and the voltage drop across the hot wire and the current in it immediately after switching on the heating circuit and again at intervals during the test period are measured and noted.

After an appropriate heating time, the heating circuit is disconnected. All measurements and recordings of the differential thermocouple are stopped. Allow time for the hot wire and test assembly to reach an equilibrium temperature and verify the uniformity and constancy of the temperature. Repeat the procedures from closing the heating circuit and power input and temperature measurements, obtaining a further measurement of the rate of rising of the temperature of the hot wire under the same conditions.

Now, from the data obtained by this technique, that is heat generated due to passing a fixed current under a fixed voltage drop through the fixed length wire, time of heating, the temperature difference between two circuits, and the separation distance between the two wires, the thermal conductivity of the refractory material is calculated.

4.5.3 Refractoriness or Pyrometric Cone Equivalent

The objective of this test is to determine the softening point of refractories by comparing the test samples (as cones) prepared from the refractory materials under test against standard pyrometric cones heated in a suitable furnace. The softening or deformation of a cone corresponds to a certain heat-work conditions that are dependent on the effects of time, temperature, and atmosphere. Hence, the test is done at a specified heating rate in a standard atmosphere to compare the temperature of softening.

First, the test refractory sample or portions of some test pieces are taken, and then by crushing and grinding the sample, a fine powder (approximately finer than 0.2 mm) is made. The magnet is used to separate out any iron particles introduced during grinding and crushing operations. To avoid excessive reduction of the fines, they are frequently removed during the process of reduction by passing the sample through the sieve and grinding of coarser particles is continued until all of the sample passes through the sieve. The powder is then mixed with alkali-free organic binder (dextrin or glue) and water. Test cones are prepared by placing the mixture in a metal mold, preferably made of brass, in the shape of truncated trigonal pyramid. The prepared shape has dimensions of 8 mm on the sides of the base, and about 25 mm high, as shown in Figure 4.3. Sufficient handling strength in the green shapes is developed by drying or by a preliminary firing at about 1000°C.

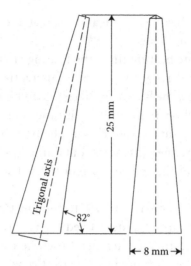

FIGURE 4.3 Schematic diagram of a pyrometric cone.

The cones made from the refractory test sample are mounted along with the standard pyrometric cones (Seger/Orton/equivalent) on a refractory round plaque with the help of a bonding material. The plaque and the bonding material must not react and affect the test and standard cones. Mounting of the test and standard cones are done with about 3 mm deep embedment in the plaque and one of the faces inclined toward the center of plaque at an angle of 82° with the horizontal. Test cones and standard cones are placed at the outer edge of the plaque and arranged in such a way to place test cones in between the standard cones. Standard cones are selected in an anticipated range, as practicable as possible.

Next the plaque containing the cone samples are placed inside a special furnace (PCE furnace) and is heated following some standard specific schedule, initially very fast, reaching about 1600°C in about 1 h. Necessary care is required to have a uniform distribution of heat and to avoid any direct flame contact with the samples and any reducing environment formation. The cones are regularly viewed to check their condition during the whole heating process through the top opening or a peep hole. At higher temperatures, the cones start to soften, and the softening temperature of a cone is marked by the bending over of the cone and the tip of the cone touching the plaque surface. Any bloating, squatting, or unequal fusion of small constituent particles is noted. Once the test cones start to soften (Figure 4.4), the heating and the experiment is stopped. The softening point of the test sample is reported with regard to the standard pyrometric

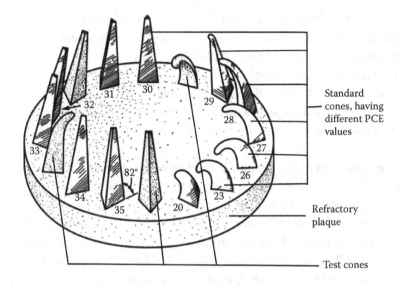

FIGURE 4.4   Schematic diagram of conditions of the pyrometric cones during the test.

cones, which is for the cone most nearly corresponds to softening behavior of the test cone. If the test cone softens in between two standard cones and approximately midway between, the softening point is reported by mentioning both the cone numbers like cone No. 35–36. If the test cone starts bending at an early cone but it does not bend down completely, or its tip does not touch the base even until a later cone, the same fact is noted.

4.6 TESTING OF THERMOMECHANICAL PROPERTIES

The evaluation of the thermomechanical properties of the refractories is of greater importance from the application points of view. Any refractory has to withstand high load at elevated temperatures and their strength evaluation is of prime importance in that condition.

4.6.1 Hot MOR

The evaluation of the modulus of rupture of refractories at elevated temperatures has become a widely accepted means to evaluate and judge the performance of the materials at service temperatures. A progressive application of force or stress is done on a specimen supported by two supports close to two ends (like a simple beam) and a center-point loading inside a furnace with uniform elevated temperature under oxidizing conditions. The load at failure is recorded to evaluate the MOR at that elevated temperature. Refractory materials will reach a semiplastic state at elevated temperatures, where Hooke's law does not apply, that is, stress is then not proportional to strain and the sample breaks down.

The rectangular bar-shaped samples with dimensions 150 mm × 25 mm × 25 mm cut from the shaped refractory products are used for this testing. Attention is focused on preparing the test pieces with smooth surfaces and clean edges. If the pressing direction is known, then the test pieces are cut in such a way that the loading direction of the testing must match with the pressing direction of the sample during shaping, and none of the other longitudinal faces of the test pieces match with the original fired surface of the brick. Test pieces are heated inside the special furnace to the specific temperature of testing and then are soaked for temperature uniformity. Next, the test pieces are loaded one after another with a constant rate of increase of stress until failure occurs. The load–stress at failure is measured and noted.

The furnace shall be (a) batch type, in which some (4 to 6) test pieces are heated to the test temperature together and tested in turn or (b) sequential type, in which the test pieces are heated to the test temperature one after another as they pass through the apparatus. In either case, the furnace shall be capable of providing the overall heating of both the bending device and the test pieces, and shall be so designed that at the moment of test the temperature distribution in the test piece is uniform within 10°C. Within the furnace one pair of lower bearing edges, made from the volume-stable refractory material, is installed with a gap of 125-mm at centers. A thrust column, containing the top bearing edge that is made from volume-stable refractory, is also extended to outside the furnace where means are provided for applying a load. The lower bearing edges and the bearing end of the support column shall have rounded bearing surfaces having about the 6-mm radius. The thrust column is maintained in a vertical alignment, and all bearing surfaces are parallel in both horizontal directions. The atmosphere inside the furnace is air (oxidizing environment). The temperature is measured by a calibrated thermocouple in the proximity of the midpoint of the tensile face of the test piece.

A heating rate of 2–10°C/min is maintained with a soaking time of 30 min at the test temperature. After the soaking period, loading is done. The rate of increase of the load is done as given in the following:

1. For a dense-shaped refractory product, $0.15 \text{ N mm}^{-2} \text{ s}^{-1}$

2. For an insulating refractory product, $0.05 \text{ N mm}^{-2} \text{ s}^{-1}$

Once a test sample is broken, the load is noted. Next the other samples are moved along the lower bearing edge and placed under the thrust column and broken as per the preceding procedure. From the sample dimensions, the gap between the supporting bearing edges and load value, hot MOR is calculated.

4.6.2 Creep

Creep can be defined as the isothermal deformation of a stressed product as a function of time. Here a test sample of given dimensions is heated under specified conditions to a given temperature, and a constant compressive load is applied to it. The deformation of the test sample, as the percent change in dimension (length) at constant temperature and load, is recorded as a function of time.

The test piece is a cylinder of 50 mm diameter and 50 mm height, with a hole of 12–13 mm diameter, extending throughout the height of the test piece, bored coaxially with the cylindrical outer surface. The top and bottom faces of the test piece must be plane and parallel by sawing (and grinding if necessary), and is perpendicular to the axis of the cylinder. The surface of the cylinder shall be free from any visible defects.

The loading device is capable of applying a load centered on the common axis of the loading column (moving one), the test piece and the supporting column (fixed column), and directed vertically along this axis at all stages of the test. The sample is rested between the loading column and the supporting column with the same common axis. A constant compressive load is applied in a downward direction from above on the piece resting directly or indirectly on a fixed base. Any deformation of the test piece is measured, generally by a dial gauge with a measurement sensitivity of 0.005 mm. Two disks, 5 mm to 10 mm thick and at least 50 mm in diameter of an appropriate refractory material compatible with the test material are placed between the test piece and the columns. The columns and disks are capable of withstanding the applied load up to the final test temperature without significant deformation. There should be no reaction between the disks and the loading system.

A vertical axis furnace, with a capacity to raise the temperature uniformly to desired test temperature by 5 K/min in air atmosphere is used for the test. During any period of constant temperature, the fluctuations of temperature must be controlled within 5 K. A central thermocouple, passing through the fixed column and the sample through the axis, is placed at the midpoint of the test piece, for measuring the temperature of the test piece at its geometric center. A control thermocouple, placed in a sheath and situated very close to the test piece, is used to control the furnace temperature. The thermocouples shall be made of platinum and platinum–rhodium wire, and shall be compatible with the final test temperature.

Precisely measured test sample is placed between the supporting and loading columns with the spacing discs, and the measuring device is adjusted to the correct setting. Next a constant compressive load is applied to the loading column at one or other of the following stages in the test:

1. At the moment when the furnace is switched on, that is, from ambient temperature.

2. After the test piece has been maintained at the test temperature for a given time (minimum 1 h, maximum 4 h).

This loading condition is to be stated in the test report. A specific load to be applied to the test piece may vary from one experiment to another, and the total load applied to the sample must include the mass of the moving column and the associated disk for any calculation. A specific load of 0.2 N/mm^2 for dense refractories and 0.05 N/mm^2 for insulating products are used. The total load used is rounded to the nearest 1 N value. For the test where the load is applied when the furnace is switched on, recording of the changes in the height of the test piece and its temperature is done at a gap of 5 min during heating and for the first hour after attaining constant temperature as indicated by the control thermocouple. After that, the changes at every 30 min intervals are to be recorded till the completion of the test.

When the load is applied to the test piece soaked at the desired constant temperature, recording of the change in height of the test piece and its temperature is done by starting with load application at a 5 min gap for the first hour and after that at every 30 min gap till the completion of the test. The standard time for testing is from 25 to 100 h. In a test where the load is applied when the furnace is switched on, the results are plotted as the percentage change in the height of the test piece as a function of temperature first till the attainment of the desired temperature and then it is plotted against the time of test at that fixed temperature.

4.6.3 Refractoriness under Load

Refractoriness under load (RUL) indicates the maximum applicable temperature of any refractory and determines the softening temperature of the refractories under a specific load indicated either by complete sagging (deforming) or breaking of the test specimen. A load of 2 kgf/cm^2 (0.2 MPa) is applied on the cylindrical sample with diameter and height, both of 50 mm. The cylindrical test sample is obtained by boring or cutting and grinding out of the central portion of the brick to be tested. The original surface of the brick should form one of the end faces of the finished test specimen. Specimens with cracks or other visible defects must not be used.

The furnace used for this testing is a specially made cylindrical electrically heated one using coke particles to conduct the high-voltage power supply and generate heat from their resistance. Packing of the coke particles is important for controlling the heating rate of the furnace. Coke particles form the outer layer of the furnace. In the inner portion, the furnace consists of a heating tube (made of corundum, magnesite, or mullite) of 100–120 mm in diameter and about 500 mm length with a wall thickness of 10–15 mm. The zone of approximately uniform temperature shall have a minimum length of 100–120 mm. A loading arrangement is done to provide a constant load of 0.2 MPa vertically to the test piece. Provision is also done for recording changes in the height of the test specimen during heating of the sample by a dial gauge and to permit it to be compressed by at least 20 mm. The setup for the test is shown in Figure 4.5.

A specific load of 0.2 MPa is applied to the test sample after it is placed in-between two rods (support rod and loading rod), generally made up of carbon or mullite. Interpose carbon plates of 5 mm thickness and above 50 mm diameter are used in between the rods and the test specimen. The dial gauge reading for measuring the dimensional change of the sample is adjusted to zero position, and then heating is started. The specific heating rate is followed as per different standard specification. As per Japanese JIS R 2209, it is 6°C per min till 1000°C and 4°C/min above 1000°C. As per Indian IS 1528—Part 2, the heating rate is 15°C/min up to 1000°C and above 1000°C at a constant rate of 8°C/min. The difference between the actual temperature rise and the scheduled rise of temperature should not vary more than 20°C at any time. The dimensional change of the sample is plotted, and a temperature versus deformation curve is obtained. The temperature is measured with an optical pyrometer, sighted or adjusted upon the bottom of a refractory tube closed at its bottom and suspended in the

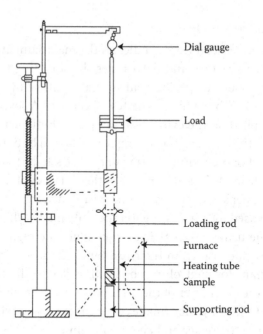

FIGURE 4.5 Schematic diagram of the setup for the RUL test.

furnace at the beginning of the test at about the middle of the test specimen. As per JIS 2209, the temperature corresponding maximum increase
in length of the test sample is marked as the apparent initial softening temperature (T1), and also the temperatures corresponding to 2% (T2) and
20% (T3) shrinkage in height of the samples are noted and the temperature
ranges (T2–T1) and (T3–T1) are calculated. As per Indian standard (IS
1528), temperature (T_a, termed as the temperature of appearance) corresponding to 0.6% deformation and temperature (T_e, termed as the temperature of the end) corresponding to 40% shrinkage is noted and reported.
In the case of premature breaking of the test specimen, actual softening
does not take place, and the temperature of breaking (T_b) is reported.

As per ASTM C 832 (reaffirmed 2015), a similar testing is termed as "thermal expansion under load." In this testing, a sample of 38 mm × 38 mm
cross section with 114 mm height is used under a load of 172 kPa stress
and a heating rate of 55 ± 5°C per hour is maintained. Continuous linear
change data is recorded in a computerized system, or manual system data
is recorded after every 55°C till 1095°C and then after every 28°C interval.
Heating is stopped when the linear expansion ceases, and the temperature
is noted. This temperature corresponds to the maximum level of expansion when the creep (deformation) rate equals to expansion rate.

4.7 TESTING FOR CORROSION RESISTANCE

Chemical attack on refractories is very common as the applications of the refractories involve contacts with corrosive solids, liquids, and gases. The corrosion from solid is very less, but that of liquid and gases are very prominent. Among different gaseous environments that a refractory encounters, carbon monoxide gas is important for refractories that are used for blast furnace applications. Again for liquid corrosion, the slag of the metallurgical sectors and glass in the glass industries are important for the refractories.

4.7.1 Testing of Resistance against Carbon Monoxide

The presence of iron oxide in the refractories, especially for fireclays, causes a disintegration effect in the CO environment and shatters the whole refractory lining. This test method compares the refractories under an accelerated exposure to CO to determine whether they can withstand the disintegrating action of CO. The test is done in an atmosphere having only CO environment, which is much higher in the concentration of CO prevailing in the actual service conditions. The results obtained by this method are used to select refractories that are resistant to CO disintegration.

A gas-tight heat chamber, heated by electrical resistance wire, is used for the test provided with a thermocouple and gas inlet and outlet openings. The chamber is also equipped with the provision for gas sampling at the outlet port and temperature controller and recorder during testing. Test samples [228 mm × 64 mm × 64 mm or 228 mm × 76 mm × 76 mm (as per ASTM C 288) or 50 mm long 30 mm diameter cylindrical sample (IS 1528 Pt 13)] with as many original surfaces as possible, are made by cutting from fired refractory shapes. For unfired shapes, a preliminary firing at around 1100°C is necessary for the test pieces before the test.

First, the heating chamber containing the test specimens is heated to an operating temperature of 495–505°C (ASTM) or 450°C (IS) in a nitrogen atmosphere. After attaining the desired temperature, the atmosphere of the chamber is changed by passing CO gas through the inlet and drained out from the outlet opening. The heating chamber should contain at least 95% CO. Carbon monoxide gas used for the test is taken from a gas cylinder or is generated from formic acid and sulfuric acid or by passing the carbon dioxide from a cylinder over charcoal heated around 1000°C in a tube furnace. The CO gas is purified by passing it through a purifying train to remove carbon dioxide, oxygen, and water vapor. Magnesium perchlorate, silica gel, or phosphorus pentoxide are also used for the removal of water vapors. A manometer and flowmeter are included in the gas train before the entrance of the gas into the furnace. A constant flow rate of CO [2 in³/h·in³ (ASTM) or 2 L/h (IS)] is maintained all through the testing. After the fixed time of testing, the CO gas flow is stopped and a fast flow of nitrogen gas is done through the furnace to flush out any remaining CO gas. Next the samples are cooled within the heating chamber in nitrogen gas environment and then taken out for inspection. Inspection is done for general discoloration, carbon deposition, cracking, and disintegration. The test is continued for a maximum of 100 h or until the test pieces disintegrate, whichever is earlier. Only the period during which the hot test pieces are exposed to the stream of carbon monoxide is considered.

Reporting of the test results is done, by mentioning the state of the test samples after testing:

1. Unaffected—when no particles spall and no cracking occurs

2. Affected—surface pop-outs, when destructive action is confined to spalls or surface pop-outs of up to 13 mm in diameter

3. Affected—cracked, when destructive action produces spalls or pop-outs greater than 1/2 in. (13 mm) in diameter, or cracking, or both

4. Destructive condition—when the specimen breaks into two or more pieces, or when hand pressure can cause breaking

4.7.2 Testing of Resistance against Liquid Corrosion

Among different liquids that affect and corrode the refractories, slag and glass are most common. So the measurement of corrosion against these liquids is necessary and important for selecting the suitable refractory for a particular application. But the application conditions of a refractory vary widely and are complex in nature. Hence, the standardization of this corrosion test is difficult to replicate in the conditions that exist in the actual application environment. Different test methods are practiced as per suitability and easiness to evaluate the corrosion of the refractory. Unfortunately, most of the testing methods for liquid corrosion are not available in the standard specifications and testing is done as per conventional or customized practice. The most commonly used and easy method for testing corrosion against a liquid is static cup method; there are dynamic methods also, namely finger test and rotary slag tester, all of which are described in the following.

4.7.2.1 Static Cup Method

In this method, a cylindrical hole is created in the central portion of a refractory cube or cuboid with retaining sufficient of the refractory wall in all the sides and the bottom of the refractory shape. Next the solidified powdered sample of the corroding material (slag or glass) is placed in the hole. Next the refractory sample with the corrosive powder is heated in a furnace to the desired temperature, generally up to the application temperature of the refractory and hold there for some prefixed period. At that test temperature, the corrosive powder will become liquid after melting and will react with the refractory and corrosion will occur along the contact surface of the refractory and the liquid. After cooling, the samples are cut through the vertical axis and the dimension of the corroded (eaten away) portion is measured. Also, any component or constituent of the corrosive liquid may enter (penetrate) the refractory but may not corrode it. In such a case, the penetration of any particular component within the refractory is measured as penetration depth. A schematic diagram of the axially cut corroded sample is shown in Figure 4.6. Also, the detailed microstructural study of the corroded portion of the samples can be done to understand the reactions that might have occurred, components of slag and refractory that have reacted and the new phases that are formed.

But this testing method is not replicating the actual conditions where the refractory surface and the corrosive liquid are in dynamic contact, and the refractory surface is always in contact with the fresh liquid. Static condition and the same fixed slag (causing saturation of slag) reduce the severity of the corrosive action and that do not represent the actual situation.

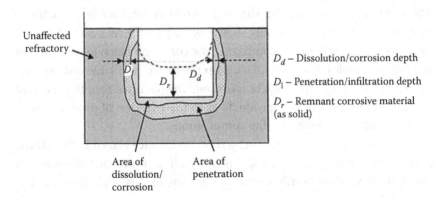

Unaffected refractory

D_d – Dissolution/corrosion depth

D_1 – Penetration/infiltration depth

D_r – Remnant corrosive material (as solid)

Area of dissolution/corrosion

Area of penetration

FIGURE 4.6 Schematic diagram of the cross section of the cup after static corrosion test.

However, through the static method, some idea about corrosion of the refractory, trend of reaction, and the reacting phases that are involved in the corrosion and the product phases that are formed, etc. are obtained. This test method may be used for comparisons purpose amongst different types of refractories against a specific corrosive liquid composition.

4.7.2.2 Finger Test (Dynamic Method)

This corrosion testing method involves of suspending small pieces of refractory samples, a bar or a cylinder (like a finger shape), in a corrosive molten liquid (slag or glass) bath. This method may also be termed as immersion method and is used when the quantity of the corrosive liquid is far more than refractory. In most of the cases, this test is done on slag samples. The refractory sample is rotated within the molten slag bath for a specific period and thus imparts a dynamic relative motion between the refractory surface and the reacting slag. Also, the refractory is facing the fresh slag, and the slag composition remains nearly unaltered (which changes for the static method as the corroded components of the refractory mix or dissolve in the limited amount of slag and change the composition) as the amount of slag is much higher compared to refractory sample. After the test, the suspending sample is taken out of the slag, allowed to cool down, cut through the cross section, and checked for dimensional loss as the measurement for corrosion. Also the penetration depth for any component of slag, if any, can be measured. Detailed microstructural studies can also be conducted, as mentioned in a static method.

4.7.2.3 Rotary Slag Test (Dynamic Method)

The rotary slag test evaluates the slag corrosion behavior of refractories in a rotating furnace, generally in the presence of a reference material. This testing method allows comparing the corrosion behavior of different refractory samples, also a standard material, under the same testing conditions against a specific slag composition. The obtained results are useful for the development of new products or in the selection of products to be used in contact with similar slag compositions.

The rotary slag tester consists of a rotating furnace placed in little tilted position, made up of a cylindrical metal shell mounted on rollers and is motor driven. A gas burner capable of heating to very high temperature, says 1750°C, is used, attached with gas and oxygen flow meters. The slag is constantly charged and renewed to maintain the original slag composition and to keep similarity as that of the application conditions. The addition of fresh slag automatically removes the already reacted molten slag present in the slag pool of the tester, and a slag flow occurs in the downward direction. The flow of the slag can also cause mechanical erosion of the refractory similar to actual application areas. The tilt angle and rotational speed of the furnace are specified and fixed as they affect the wear rate.

Test specimens of length 228 (230) mm and cross section and shape (as shown in Figure 4.7) are used for the testing with slag contact face as the original molded surface. One or more reference samples are included in each test run along with the test samples. A number of test samples, six or more, are arranged to constitute the test lining. Suitable granular refractory or castable is used behind the test lining to hold the test samples with the cylindrical shell. At both the ends, the inert material lining is given to protect the shell from liquid slag. The whole assembly is then held in place by retaining rings bolted to each end of the shell. The shell, with the test specimens, is then placed in its cradle and linkage is made to the driving motor. The gas-oxygen torch mounting is adjusted for firing axially through the furnace. Ground and shaped (by extrusion or pressing) slag

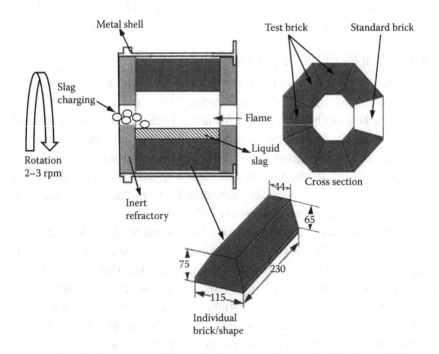

FIGURE 4.7   Schematic diagram of the rotary slag corrosion tester, including its cross section and the shape and size of the refractory test sample.

pellets are fed into the slag tester and counted to determine the number of pellets charged during the test to calculate and control the slag flow rate.

The furnace is typically tilted ~3° axially down toward the burner end. The furnace, preheated by the gas-oxygen torch is fired to a temperature to melt the slag pellets. After reaching the desired temperature, soaking for 30 min is done. The molten slag washes over the lining and drips from the lower end of the furnace in front of the burner. The furnace rotates at a constant speed of 2–3 rpm and an oxidizing atmosphere is maintained. This rotation imparts the dynamic motion between the slag and the refractory. During the test, slag layer temperature is measured by the optical pyrometer. Regular feeding of slag pellets is done to make fresh contact of slag with the refractories, and the whole process runs for about 5 h (depending on the quality of the refractory). After the stipulated period, the firing and the rotating motor is stopped. Next, the furnace is tilted to a vertical position to remove all the remaining slag. After cooling, the furnace is disassembled, and the refractories are checked through the length perpendicular to and at the center of the slag contact face. Measurement of the dimensions for corrosion, penetration, is taken after cutting the samples and microstructural studies, if required, are done as mentioned earlier.

4.8 TESTING OF ABRASION RESISTANCE

This testing method measures the resistance of a refractory material against abrasion. The abrasion of refractory is defined as the surface wear caused by the mechanical action of moving solids. The testing method determines the volume of the material abraded from a flat surface of a test piece placed at right angles to a nozzle through which of size-graded abrading grains are blasted by compressed air at a specific pressure. Mostly, all the different standards have the same concept of measurement, and only the individual testing parameters are different.

The test system requires an abrasion tester consisting of a Venturi blast assembly of an air blast gun and a nozzle. The nozzle directs the abrading grains onto the test piece under compressed air. There is also a feed mechanism, capable of supplying a fixed amount of abrasive grains to the blast assembly at a specific time. A tightly sealed test chamber is used with a door to permit ready access for mounting and removing the test pieces. A manometer is used to measure the pressure inside the chamber during the test with a vacuum gauge to check the pressure at the entry point for the abrasive grains on the blast assembly. Silicon carbide abrasive grains of size between 0.85 and 0.6 mm amounting 800 g and 0.6–0.3 mm amounting to 200 g (total 1000 g) is used for testing.

The samples of dimension 100 mm × 100 mm × 25 mm are cut from refractory bricks or shapes in such a way so that one of the square faces of each test piece is an original surface.

Next, the test pieces are dried to constant weight, and its bulk density is measured. Then each piece is placed in the test chamber with the square face (original molded surface) facing the nozzle at a distance of 203 mm from the nozzle mouth. Compressed air supply with regulated pressure at 450 kPa is used to maintain a chamber pressure of 310 kPa. After the desired level of pressure is obtained in the test chamber and compressed air system, the feed mechanism is connected to the blast assembly and the total abrasive grains are blasted on the sample for 450 s. After the test, the weight of the sample was again measured and the abrasion loss (A) is calculated as

$$A = \text{Weight loss/Bulk density (unit } cm^3).$$

4.9 TESTING OF THERMAL SHOCK RESISTANCE

Thermal shock or spalling is the cracking or fracture of the refractory product caused by differential expansion due to thermal shock, a steep temperature gradient, a crystalline conversion, or a change in composition near the hot face. For qualitative measurement, expressed in the number of cycles that a refractory material can withstand, different techniques may be used to determine the thermal shock (spalling) resistance. There is also some quantitative measurement technique of thermal shock resistance, measured as the loss of strength or loss of Young's modulus of any sample due to some specific number of thermal cycles. The popular methods for determining the thermal shock resistance are described in the following.

4.9.1 Water Quenching Method

This is a qualitative measurement of thermal shock. A refractory test specimen of standard brick dimension 230 mm × 115 mm × 75 mm is taken. An electric heating furnace with controlling facility to maintain the temperature within 10°C is used. A water tank, which can maintain constant water flow is used for quenching or cooling the heated specimen.

The test specimen is dried at 110°C to constant weight, and the weight is taken. Next the test specimen is inserted into the furnace chamber, maintaining a temperature of 1300°C, up to a depth of 50 mm length-wise. Any gap is be filled up by light fireclay inserts and asbestos. After insertion of the test specimen in the furnace, the temperature is again raised to 1300°C and the specimen is kept at 1300°C for 10 min. After heating, the specimen is taken out from the furnace, and the heated end is dipped into the water tank to a depth of 50 mm (the heated part only). The water tank is connected to running water at ambient temperature with a flow rate of 7 L/min. The test specimen is kept in the water for 5 min and then taken out and kept in air for 5 min. This heating for 10 min and then cooling in water for 5 min and air for 5 min completes one thermal cycle. This cycle of heating and cooling of the specimen is repeated, and any weight loss of sample is checked after each cooling. When there is a weight loss of 20% of the specimen, lost by flaking off, the test is stopped, and the number of the cycle just before the 20% loss is reported as the number of cycles that the specimen can withstand.

4.9.2 Small Prism Method

This is also a qualitative measurement of thermal shock resistance of a refractory sample. Test pieces are cut or ground to the shape of prisms 75 mm high with a square base of 50 mm (or rings of 50 mm height from sleeves, nozzles). A muffle or semimuffle type electrically heated furnace is used for the purpose of heating attached to a thermocouple for measuring temperature.

Test samples are placed in the furnace in the cold condition. Heating is done to reach the desired temperature, say 1000°C, in about 3 h time. First, the sample is soaked for 30 min at that temperature for uniformity of temperature in the sample and then the test pieces are taken out from the furnace. Hot samples are then placed on their square face over a brick floor having nearly no air flow. The test samples are cooled in air for 10 min and then again placed in the furnace, maintained at that desired temperature. One heating and one cooling step complete a thermal cycle. Next each heating and cooling operation will be for 10 min only. After each cooling period, the sample is examined for any crack formation on the surface (visual observation). Once the crack appears on the sample surface, the test is stopped and the number of the cycles during which the cracks first appear is reported.

4.9.3 Deterioration in Property after Thermal Shock

This test method determines the strength loss or reduction in continuity, or both, of prism-shaped test samples after a certain numbers of thermal cycling. The strength loss is measured by measuring the cold modulus of rupture (MOR) of the samples before and after thermal shocks. Also, the reduction in structural continuity is estimated by the difference in sonic velocity before and after thermal cycles. This indicates the ability of the refractory test piece to withstand the stress generated by sudden changes in temperature, from the heating temperature.

Visually crack- and flaw-free test samples, 10 in number from two different bricks or shapes, with dimensions 150 mm × 25 mm × 25 mm and having, at least, one original surface in each sample, are used for this testing. An electrically heated furnace that can heat and maintain 1200°C with temperature recovery time of less than 5 min, a standard mechanical or hydraulic compression testing machine, and a sonic velocity machine are the apparatus required for this testing.

First, the sonic velocity along the length of each test specimen is measured and next the cold modulus of rupture, using three-point loading bending setup is determined. Then the furnace is preheated to the test temperature of 1200°C, and the test specimens are placed into the furnace spanning the setter brick and kept them for 10–15 min. Then, the samples are taken out and cooled for 10–15 min while spanning the setter brick in ambient air. This one heating and one cooling period is considered as one full cycle. A total of five such complete cycles are conducted and each heating cycle is considered once the furnace starts maintaining the desired temperature after recovery. After thermal cycles, the sonic velocity of each specimen is measured along the length and cold modulus of rupture is tested. The percent sonic velocity loss of each specimen is calculated as

$$\frac{(V_i - V_f) \times 100}{V_i}$$

where V_i is the initial sonic velocity of each specimen (m/s) and V_f = sonic velocity of each specimen after thermal cycles (m/s). Also, the percent loss in modulus of rupture strength of the specimen is calculated as

$$\frac{(M_i - M_f) \times 100}{M_i}$$

where M_i is the average cold modulus of rupture strength of the original specimens (MPa) and M_f is the average cold modulus of rupture strength of the specimen after thermal cycling (MPa).

4.10 SUMMARY

A quantitative estimation of the properties of refractories is done by various testing methods.

Testing methods for any single property may vary depending on the specific testing standard followed for testing.

The results of the same property testing of the same material may differ with sample size and mode of testing, and the rate of certain operation involved in testing may differ in different standard specifications.

Refractories, being ceramic materials, have preexisting pores and cracks, result in non-uniformity of properties. Hence, the average data of few samples is to be represented by each type of testing to get a predictable behavior of the material during use.

Different countries or zones of the globe have different standard testing methods and specifications.

Bulk density, apparent porosity, apparent specific gravity, and water absorption values can be obtained from a single experiment, which can be conducted by two different methods, namely boiling method (non-hydraulic samples) and vacuum method.

Specific gravity or true density is measured using powdered samples by pycnometric method.

Mechanical strength measurements both at ambient and elevated temperatures are dependent on sample size and loading rate, specification followed to measure them, etc. The results may differ for the same quality of the refractory due to these, and so all these parameters are to be mentioned in the report.

For thermal properties, thermal expansion is measured by using a dilatometer. A vitreous silica-based system is used up to a temperature of 1150°C and for higher temperatures alumina based dilatometers are used. Thermal conductivity is measured by calorimetric or hot wire methods, and well precaution is required to be taken to prevent any heat loss and error in the results.

Corrosion testing can be done by various methods but the simple techniques are far from reality and application environment. Rotary slag tester approaches to the close approximation of the actual applications but still have issues like the rotation of refractory, non-continuous contact with slag, etc.

Thermal shock resistance can be measured by both qualitative and quantitative methods.

QUESTIONS AND ASSIGNMENTS

1. Why do we need a standard specification for measuring the properties?

2. Describe in detail how bulk density and apparent porosities are measured.

3. Why do we need to consider the liquid density for calculating bulk density but not for apparent porosity when a liquid other than water is used?

4. How is true specific gravity measured?

5. How can closed porosity be measured?

6. Describe the difference between the different thermomechanical property measurements.

7. Describe the difference between different test methods for liquid corrosion resistances.

8. How can the refractoriness of an unknown sample be measured?

9. Describe the difference between different test methods for thermal shock resistances.

10. Describe the measurement technique of creep.

11. Detail the testing method for thermal expansion.

12. How is carbon monoxide disintegration test done?

13. What are the drawbacks of static cup method for liquid corrosion test?

14. What are the different dynamic slag corrosion tests? Describe any one of the processes in detail methods.

BIBLIOGRAPHY

1. A. Rashid Chesti, *Refractories: Manufacture, Properties and Applications*, Prentice-Hall of India, New Delhi, India, 1986.
2. W. David Kingery, H. K. Bowen, and D. R. Uhlmann, *Introduction to Ceramics*, 2nd edn., John Wiley and Sons Inc., New York, 1976.
3. F. Singer and S. S. Singer, *Industrial Ceramics*, Springer, Berlin, 1963.
4. J. H. Chesters, *Refractories—Production and Properties*, Woodhead Publishing Ltd., Cambridge, UK, 2006.

5. P. P. Budnikov, *The Technology of Ceramics and Refractories*, 4th edn., Translated by E. Arnold, *Scripta Technica*, The MIT Press, Cambridge, MA, 2003.
6. F. H. Norton, *Refractories*, 4th edn., McGraw-Hill, New York, 1968.
7. C. A. Schacht, *Refractories Handbook*, CRC Press, Boca Raton, FL, 2004.
8. *Harbison-Walker Handbook of Refractory Practice*, Harbison-Walker, PA, 2005.
9. S. C. Carniglia and G. L. Barna, *Handbook of Industrial Refractories Technology: Principles, Types, Properties, and Applications*, Noyes Publications, Saddle River, NJ, 1992.
10. *Standard Test Methods for Apparent Porosity, Liquid Absorption, Apparent Specific Gravity, and Bulk Density of Refractory Shapes by Vacuum Pressure*, ASTM C830-00, 2011.
11. *Standard Test Methods for Apparent Porosity, Water Absorption, Apparent Specific Gravity, and Bulk Density of Burned Refractory Brick and Shapes by Boiling Water*, ASTM C20-00, 2015.
12. *Standard Test Methods for Cold Crushing Strength and Modulus of Rupture of Refractories*, ASTM C133-97, 2015.
13. *Standard Test Method for Modulus of Rupture of Refractory Materials at Elevated Temperatures*, ASTM C583-15, 2015.
14. *Standard Test Method for Measuring Thermal Expansion and Creep of Refractories under Load*, ASTM C832-00, 2015.
15. *Standard Test Method for Thermal Conductivity of Refractories by Hot Wire (Platinum Resistance Thermometer Technique)*, ASTM C1113/C1113M-09, 2013.
16. *Standard Test Method for Thermal Conductivity of Refractories*, ASTM C201-93, 2013.
17. *Standard Test Method for Pyrometric Cone Equivalent (PCE) of Fireclay and High Alumina Refractory Materials*, ASTM C24-09, 2013.
18. *Standard Test Method for Abrasion Resistance of Refractory Materials at Room Temperature*, C704/C704M-15, 2015.
19. *Standard Test Method for Disintegration of Refractories in an Atmosphere of Carbon Monoxide*, ASTM C288-87, 2014.
20. *Standard Test Method for True Specific Gravity of Refractory Materials by Water Immersion*, ASTM C135-96, 2015.
21. *Standard Test Method for Rotary Slag Testing of Refractory Materials*, ASTM C874-11a, 2011.
22. *Methods of Sampling and Physical Tests for Refractory Materials, Determination of Cold Crushing Strength of Dense Shaped Refractories Products*, Indian Standard Specification IS 1528—Part IV, 2012.
23. *Methods of Sampling and Physical Tests for Refractory Materials, Method for Determination of Modulus of Rupture at Ambient Temperature of Dense and Insulating Shaped Refractory Products*, Indian Standard Specification IS 1528—Part 5, 2007.

24. *Methods of Sampling and Physical Tests for Refractory Materials, Determination of Pyrometric Cone Equivalent (PCE) or Softening Point,* Indian Standard Specification IS 1528—Part 1, 2010.

25. *Methods of Sampling and Physical Tests for Refractory Materials, Determination of Refractoriness under Load,* Indian Standard Specification IS 1528—Part 2, 2011.

26. *Methods of Sampling and Physical Tests for Refractory Materials, Determination of Spalling Resistance,* Indian Standard Specification IS 1528—Part 3, 2010.

27. *Methods of Sampling and Physical Tests for Refractory Materials, Determination of Permanent Linear Change after Reheating for Shaped Insulating and Dense Refractories,* Indian Standard Specification IS 1528—Part 6, 2010.

28. *Methods of Sampling and Physical Tests for Refractory Materials, Determination of Apparent Porosity,* Indian Standard Specification IS 1528—Part 8, 1974.

29. *Methods of Sampling and Physical Tests for Refractory Materials, Determination of True Density,* Indian Standard Specification IS 1528—Part 9, 2007.

30. *Methods of Sampling and Physical Tests for Refractory Materials, Method for Determination of Bulk Density and True Porosity of Shaped Insulating Refractory Products,* Indian Standard Specification IS 1528—Part 12, 2007.

31. *Methods of Sampling and Physical Tests for Refractory Materials, Determination of Resistance to Carbon Monoxide,* Indian Standard Specification IS 1528—Part 13, 2007.

32. *Methods of Sampling and Physical Tests for Refractory Materials, Method for Determination of Bulk Density, Apparent Porosity and True Porosity of Dense Shaped Refractory Products,* Indian Standard Specification IS 1528—Part 15, 2007.

CHAPTER 5

Silica Refractories

5.1 INTRODUCTION

Silica is the name given to a specific compound composed of silicon and oxygen, the two most abundant elements in the earth's crust. Hence silica, the only compound of these two elements, is a very common and one of the most commonly available oxide on the earth's crust. Silica is found in nature commonly in the crystalline form and rarely in an amorphous state. It is composed of one atom of silicon and two atoms of oxygen, giving rise to the chemical formula SiO_2. Quartz is the only form of silica that is thermodynamically stable in the atmospheric conditions, and so all the uncombined free form of silica present in the crust is available as quartz and is found in quartzite, sand, flint, and ganister. Quartzite is the most commonly available form of quartz and used as the major raw material for manufacturing silica refractories. The raw material must have a minimum amount of impurities like Al_2O_3, Fe_2O_3, and TiO_2 that greatly reduce the liquidus temperature and restricts high-temperature applications.

Silica refractories are those materials that contain about >93% SiO_2, with a minor amount of other oxides as additives and impurities, namely lime (CaO), alumina (Al_2O_3), and iron oxide (Fe_2O_3). Silica is acidic in character, readily reacts with alkali and alkaline earth oxides, and so silica refractories are also acidic in nature. In general, two major classes of silica, refractories are important, namely super-duty silica refractories with very high purity (impurity content Al_2O_3 + Fe_2O_3 ~0.5%) and high-duty refractories, containing impurities in the range of 0.5–2 wt%. As per historical information, silica refractories were first produced in the United Kingdom in 1822 from Ganister (carboniferous sandstone) or so called Dinas sand. For this reason, in some of the countries, silica refractories are also called dinas.

5.2 RAW MATERIALS AND SOURCES

The natural sources of silica are widely and abundantly available all over the world and are used for making silica refractories. Amongst them, quartz is most abundant and important. It is found in almost every type of rock: igneous, metamorphic, and sedimentary. Quartz is particularly abundant in sedimentary rocks as it is highly resistant to breakdown by the physical and chemical processes of weathering. Quartz is present nearly in all mining operations, in the host rock, in the ore, as well as in the soil and surface materials called the overburden.

Silica occurs in a variety of crystalline polymorphic forms, for example, quartz, tridymite, and cristobalite and also as an undercooled melt called quartz glass. Each of the polymorphic forms has a high and low temperature variations, which can transform reversibly. The crystal structure of the polymorphic forms of silica differs significantly and the transformation from one form to other is associated with a distinct change in specific gravity. These changes are of great importance during heating and cooling of silica refractories due to a corresponding change in volume, which may result in cracking and breaking of the shapes.

The polymorphic forms of silica are temperature dependent and one form changes to other on reaching a specific temperature. These changes are sluggish in nature and takes a long time to convert from one form to another due to bond breaking and reconstruction of another crystallographic structure. These changes are termed as reconstructive transformations (conversion). Again the low- and high-temperature variations of each polymorphic forms are also temperature-dependent, but as the change is only associated with little orientational changes of the structure, these transformations are very rapid and spontaneous in nature, once the desired temperature is reached. The changes are termed as displacive transformations (inversion). As per thermodynamic stability, the principal crystalline forms of silica are quartz (trigonal and hexagonal, stable up to 870°C), tridymite (hexagonal, stable from 870°C to 1470°C), and cristobalite (cubic, stable from 1470°C to 1723°C, the melting point). Vitreous silica is a metastable phase in solid form and has relatively random network structure as that of a liquid, "frozen in" by undercooling. Table 5.1 shows the details of the transformations that occur in silica.

TABLE 5.1   Details of the Crystallographic Change of Silica

Transformation Temperature (°C)	Phase Change	Specific Gravity	Volume Changes (%)	Crystal System Change
117–163	$\alpha \leftrightarrow \beta_1 \leftrightarrow \beta_2$ tridymite	2.26 ↔ 2.27	+0.5	Rhombic ↔ hexagonal ↔ hexagonal
220–280	$\alpha \leftrightarrow \beta_2$ cristobalite	2.33 ↔ 2.21	2.0 ↔ 2.8	Tetragonal ↔ cubic
573	$\alpha \leftrightarrow \beta$ quartz	2.65 ↔ 2.49	0.86 ↔ 1.3	Trigonal ↔ hexagonal
870	β quartz ↔ β_2 tridymite	2.49 ↔ 2.27	14.4	Hexagonal ↔ hexagonal
1250	β quartz ↔ β cristobalite	2.49 ↔ 2.21	~17.4	Hexagonal ↔ cubic
1470	β_2 tridymite ↔ β cristobalite	2.27 ↔ 2.21	~3	Hexagonal ↔ cubic
1713	β cristobalite ↔ liquid			

5.3 BRIEF OF MANUFACTURING TECHNIQUES

The selection of a proper raw material and its firing process are important for the silica refractories such that the degree of quartz transformation to the desired form is suitable for the intended application. As quartz, stable only up to 870°C, is the naturally occurring form of silica and polymorphic change from quartz to tridymite or cristoballite (high temperature stable) phases is associated with a very high volume changes, the amount of free quartz in the fired products must be minimum. Otherwise, free quartz will transform to the thermodynamically stable form of the application temperature during use, causing volumetric changes, and cracking and shattering of the refractory structure. Also, the polymorphic form of the fired silica refractory must match with the thermodynamically stable form at the temperature level of targeted applications.

The common raw material for silica refractory is naturally occurring quartzite, which must meet the requirements to achieve optimum brick properties. When high temperature application is the main criteria for silica refractory, then the quartzite used must have a high chemical purity, with the total impurity <0.5 wt%. For other applications, quartzites of ~95% purity are acceptable. Impurities like Al_2O_3, Fe_2O_3, TiO_2, and alkalis form low melting liquid phases and restrict the high-temperature applications.

For making the silica refractory, quartzite is first washed to remove associated clayey minerals and dust, then crushed, ground, and screened to the various grain fractions. The individual fractions are combined in predetermined proportions according to the required application and properties. In most cases, muller, pan, or counterflow mixers are used for mixing silica refractories, and different fraction sizes, namely coarse, medium, and fines are mixed. Bonding of silica refractories is achieved by the addition of milk of lime (hydrated lime) about up to 3 wt%. This lime acts as a mineralizer and accelerates the formation of desired tridymite or cristoballite phase. Some more compounds such as iron oxide, borax, magnesium oxide, barium oxide and fluorides, carbonates, phosphates of sodium, lithium, and potassium also act as mineralizers. Alkalis affect the liquidus temperature very strongly. Hence, their use as mineralizers requires very strict quantity control and compositional analysis. These mineralizers are added to the silica refractory mix in the mixer machine. Also green binder, like cellulose, sulfate lye, molasses, etc., is added to provide green (dried) strength of the refractories after shaping (pressing). The uniform distribution and mixing of these additions in the green refractory mixture ensure the uniform and improved properties of the fired refractories. The addition of zircon and silicon carbide are also done during mixing for special cases where increased resistance to abrasion and high thermal conductivity are required in the fired refractories, respectively.

Moisture is added to the mixture to make a semidry mix. It acts as a plasticizer for the mixture and helps to provide and retain the shape. The amount of moisture to be added depends on the shaping process. Table 5.2 gives an indicative idea of the amount of moisture used for different shaping processes. Higher moisture content may increase the chance of slumping of the shape after shaping and increased the probability of cracking during drying due to higher removal water vapor. Again lower moisture content demands higher pressing pressure. Low-pressure shaping processes, like hand molding, are employed for making shapes with critical dimensions and much bigger sizes that are difficult to attain in machines like in hydraulic presses. But low pressure results in low and non-uniform density and

TABLE 5.2 Variation of Moisture Requirement with Shaping Process

Shaping Process	Moisture Level (%)
Hand moulding	8–10
Pneumatic ramming	6–7
Screw friction pressing	5–6
Toggle pressing	5–6
Hydraulic pressing	4–5

strength values in the refractories. On the other hand, pressing is advantageous for uniformity and improved properties with much higher productivity. But very high pressing pressure results in high compactness in the green shape and is disadvantageous for silica refractories, as it provides an insufficient gap for the volumetric expansions that are associated with the polymorphic phase transformations of silica and may cause cracking.

After pressing, the shapes are dried to remove the physically absorbed (added) moisture and drying time depends on the shaping process. Drying is done up to a maximum temperature of 150–200°C using the excess heat of flue gas emerging from the firing kiln. For hydraulic pressed products, drying time is about 24–30 h whereas for hand-mold shapes, containing a high amount of moisture, drying time is up to 100 h; slow drying for long duration is required to avoid any crack formation due to sudden and excessive removal of vapor.

The firing of silica refractories requires special attention due to its polymorphic changes during heating. For this reason, the firing is done mostly in batch types of kilns with a long firing schedule though they are less heat efficient. Continuous firing kilns require exceptionally long preheating and cooling zones to accommodate the slow heating and cooling rates to take care of the polymorphic changes, especially the quartz transformations. The $\alpha \leftrightarrow \beta$ quartz transformation, both during heating and cooling (between 550°C and 600°C), requires very slow rate to structurally accommodate the sudden and instantaneous volume change that may generate the crack. A tentative heating and cooling schedule practiced in industry for silica refractory firing in a batch fired kiln is given in Table 5.3.

TABLE 5.3   Details of the Firing Schedule of Silica Refractory in a Batch Type Kiln

Heating		Cooling	
Temperature (°C)	Period (h)	Temperature (°C)	Period (h)
R.T.–500	24	**Close Condition**	
500–650	15	1430–800	22
650–900	17	800–600	16
900–1100	10	600–300	30
1100–1300	25	300–150	30
1300–1350	12		
1350–1410	30	**Open Condition**	
1410–1430/1480	20–24	300–150	24
Holding at			
1430/1480	48–72		

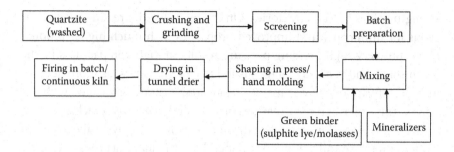

FIGURE 5.1   Manufacturing process for silica refractory.

The firing temperature of silica refractories varies between 1420°C and 1500°C depending upon the desired phase in the final fired refractories. For the applications where tridymite phase is stable, firing is done between 1420°C and 1430°C, to maximize the tridymite phase formation. For high-temperature applications of silica refractories where cristobalite phase is stable, firing is done between 1480°C and 1500°C to maximize the cristobalite phase formation. It is necessary to maintain a carefully planned time temperature schedule for getting a strong, well-bonded fired refractory with the desired polymorphic form. In general, during firing, the net linear growth of silica refractories is about 4%, and sufficient internal gaps are required within the shapes to allow such expansion. This growth is less than the actual calculated values, because of the presence of the pores that accommodate the expansion within themselves. A schematic diagram for manufacturing of silica refractories is shown in Figure 5.1.

5.4 ACTION OF MINERALIZER

The chemical compounds added to accelerate and stabilize the desired mineral phase (of silica refractory) are called mineralizers. They help to mineralize the silica to a specific desired mineral phase. Mainly, lime (CaO) in the range of 2–3 wt% (added as hydrated lime) is used for making cristobalite-based silica refractories and lime ~2 wt% and iron oxide ~0.5 wt% is used to stabilize the tridymite phase. There is a well-established concept for the formation and stabilization of cristobalite phase due to the addition of lime, as proposed by Dale, and named as Dale's theory. But for tridymite formation, such concept or theory is yet to be established.

As per Dale's theory, hydrated lime, the source of lime, loses its physical moisture within 200°C and at around 400°C, it starts decomposing to form anhydrous lime. Increasing temperature to about 800°C initiates the reaction between the fine and nascent lime with and fine silica particles in the matrix phase of the refractories and increases the bonding within matrix phase and an increase in strength. The reaction produces $2CaO\ SiO_2$ and little free $CaO\ SiO_2$ phases. Further increase in temperature increases the reaction of fine silica with the Ca-silicate phases and at about 1250–1300°C liquid phase starts forming in the $CaO–SiO_2$ system in the presence of other impurities like Fe_2O_3, Al_2O_3, TiO_2, etc. This liquid reacts with the surfaces of the large quartz grains and dissolves the silica from the surface. More of silica is converted (dissolved) into the liquid phase as temperature is further increased and the silica grains get dissolved. After a certain time, the liquid is saturated with silica and then silica will crystallize out from the supersaturated liquid phase and will crystallize as cristobalite, as per temperature conditions. The basic mechanisms involve the dissolution of quartz in a $CaO–SiO_2$ liquid and precipitation (crystallization) of cristobalite crystals (particles) from the liquid. This conversion of quartz to cristobalite in the presence of lime is much faster than the direct transformation with the effect of heat only, which is very slow and sluggish in nature.

5.5 CLASSIFICATION AND PROPERTIES OF SILICA BRICKS

Silica refractories are classified mainly into two types depending on the purity or impurity content. The super-duty silica refractories are about 97% pure and contain impurity (other than CaO, which is additive) to a maximum of 0.5%. The impurities like Al_2O_3, Fe_2O_3, and TiO_2 are responsible for low-temperature liquid phase formation in silica and, in general, they are termed as flux factor in silica refractories. The other type is general-purpose silica refractory, which is about 94% pure and has impurity level up to about 2.5%. There is also a type of silica called semisilica refractory containing about 65%–80% silica, but they come under fireclay refractories.

The main features of silica refractories are as follows:

- Low price

- Relatively low density and specific gravity

- High strength even at temperatures close to melting point (PCE)

- Nearly no shrinkage even after prolonged use

- Very high corrosion resistance against acidic liquids

- High thermal expansion at lower temperatures and low thermal expansion at high temperatures

The fired silica brick contains the crystalline forms of silica, mainly cristobalite or tridymite and little amount of unconverted and unwanted residual quartz. The additive and impurity phases present in the composition remain in the matrix as very small quantities of calcium ferrite, hematite, magnetite, alumino-silicate, etc. depending on the mineralizers used and impurities present. These minute amount of crystalline phases are responsible for the coloration and spot formation on the fired products. Silica refractories with the identical chemical composition can have differing mineralogical compositions, and this can cause quite a different behaviour during use. Therefore, it is not always sufficient to evaluate silica bricks solely by their chemical composition but essentially the degree of transformation of quartz (or the residual quartz content) and the final phases and their content in the fired refractories are important.

Free quartz present in a fired silica refractory is termed as residual quartz (RQ) and for any application, a higher RQ value is detrimental. Hence, the determination of RQ value for any silica refractory is essential. This can easily be determined by the quantitative phase analysis study through x-ray diffraction techniques. Also an accurate determination of specific gravity of the fired product gives a good idea about the RQ content. A high RQ value results in instantaneous volumetric changes during temperature change at 573°C due to α to β quartz inversion and also will convert to equilibrium-stable tridymite or cristobalite phases depending on the application temperature with huge volumetric expansions. These expansions may result in cracking and collapse of the refractory structure. An RQ value of less than 10% is essential. During the use of the silica refractory, conversion of the residual quartz occurs at high temperatures and RQ value reduces with prolonged heating or with increasing number of heating cycles.

Silica refractories are most important for their acid resistance properties. Silica remains unaffected by any acidic conditions and retains its structural integrity except for hydrofluoric acid and phosphoric acid above 400°C. The basic material like compounds of alkalis and alkaline earth elements attack silica particularly at high temperatures and form low-temperature fusible silicate compounds. So silica refractories are never used in any basic environment.

Heating up and cooling down of silica refractories from room temperature to 600°C needs special attention for their high thermal expansion values in addition to chances of cracking and disintegration. Sudden changes in length are caused by the transformation behavior of the space lattice of silica associated with the structural changes with increasing temperature.

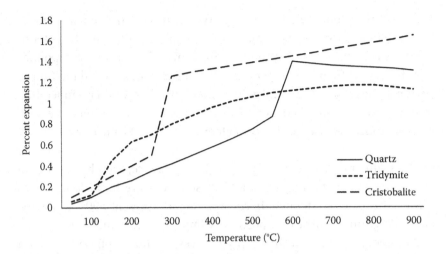

FIGURE 5.2   Thermal expansion values of different crystallographic forms of silica.

Quartz shows such a transformation at 573°C, tridymite at 117°C and 163°C, and cristobalite between 220°C and 280°C. It is also to be noted in particular that the thermal expansion value of cristobalite is considerably greater than that of the tridymite. The thermal expansion behavior of the different crystallographic forms of silica is shown against temperature in Figure 5.2. Due to these phase changes and high thermal expansion values, the thermal shock resistance of silica refractories up to 600°C is low. However, when the temperature remains above 600°C, the thermal shock resistance of silica refractories is good.

The most important characteristic of silica refractories is their refractoriness under load value, which approaches very close to that of the fusion point. No other refractory material shows such a high RUL value, close to its PCE. These two values are very close, especially for the silica refractories having a little amount of impurity. This is due to the low amount of liquid phase formation. Again whatever liquid phases are formed, they are very high silica containing liquids and have a very high viscosity. Hence, deformation under load is negligible. Thus, the refractory has nearly no deformation till the temperature close to its fusion point and has very high RUL values.

5.6 EFFECT OF IMPURITIES ON PHASE DIAGRAMS

Impurities present in the raw materials react with the silica refractories during firing of the brick and also during use. Again chemicals and ions from the environments and corrosive agents may react with the refractory and affect the properties. These impurity ions react with the main refractory system and form compounds with a completely different character or affect the high-temperature properties by forming low melting compounds or reducing the liquidus temperature. The presence of a second ion (impurity) in a pure system starts form ing a liquid phase at a lower temperature from the eutectic, peritectic, or solidus temperature, sometimes at a temperature much lower than the fusion temperature of the pure system.

For silica refractories, the main secondary oxides phases present are CaO (as mineralizer), Al_2O_3, Fe_2O_3, TiO_2, etc. Hence, the phase diagram of the systems containing silica and these oxides are important. But as silica is the major component in silica refractory (present >90% level), the phase diagram of silica rich portion is important for silica refractories. The presence of alumina drastically reduces the liquid phase formation temperature to 1587°C from a melting point of 1713–1723°C (Figure 5.3a). There is a sharp fall in liquidus temperature, and the eutectic is at a composition of ~5 mol% Al_2O_3. Again increasing the amount of CaO shows (Figure 5.3b) the formation of a eutectic at 1650°C with a CaO content of ~7 mol% and then a further increase in CaO forms an immiscible liquid. But the phase diagram shows that any minute presence of CaO in silica causes liquid phase from and above 1430°C, which is relatively low compared to its application temperatures. At that temperature, the CaO-containing silica composition remains as a mixture of tridymite phase as solid phase and a liquid phase, whose composition and amount vary with temperature. Above 1470°C, the tridymite phase converts to cristobalite and the mixture then changes as cristobalite and liquid. Hence in a pure silica system, liquid phase will start at 1430°C in the presence of CaO. The presence of TiO_2 also reduces (Figure 5.3c) the liquidus temperature drastically, and liquid phase starts forming from 1550°C, the eutectic temperature. The presence of FeO shows a similar behavior as observed for CaO (Figure 5.3d); liquid phase starts forming from the eutectic temperature of 1685°C having a eutectic composition of ~4 mol% FeO and 96 mol% SiO_2. But for a higher amount of FeO liquid phase starts forming from about 1189°C. Initially, the liquid phase is in combination with tridymite phase and at higher temperatures, with cristobalite phase after conversion of tridymite to cristobalite.

Mainly, the reduction in liquid phase formation temperature in the presence of impurities is most detrimental for silica refractories as the liquid phase formation strongly reduces the thermomechanical properties. Also, the corrosion properties are affected as liquid reacts much faster and

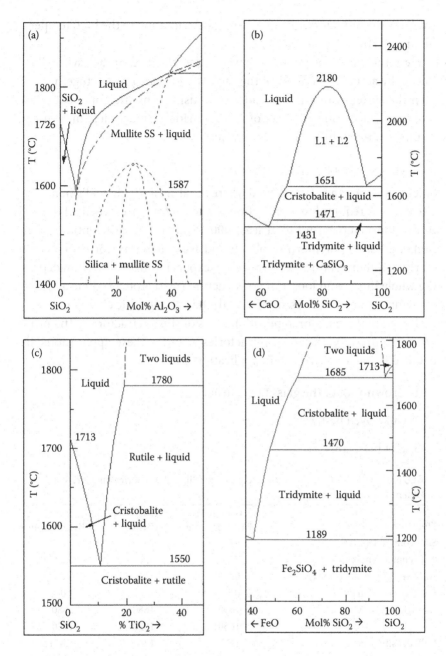

FIGURE 5.3 Phase diagrams of silica with different impurity oxides: (a) Al_2O_3, (b) CaO, (c) TiO_2, and (d) FeO.

corrodes the refractory. Overall there is deterioration in the high temperature properties.

Here the effects of impurity ions are described separately with silica. But in the actual case, many of the impurity ions are present together and then the system can only be understood using a multicomponent phase diagram. The combined effect of the impurities is much detrimental and results in a much inferior refractory quality.

5.7 MAIN APPLICATION AREAS

Silica refractories are mostly used where the atmosphere is acidic in nature. Great care is required for application of silica refractories when it is heated from room temperature to at least 600°C due to the differential expansion of different polymorphic phases and associated transformations with increasing temperature. Allowance for expansion has to be provided for the whole lining and loosening of structure (by tie rods) is done at different temperature ranges associated with the polymorphic changes.

There are three major application areas of silica refractories. The properties required for the silica refractories used for these applications are detailed in Table 5.4. The main application areas are

1. Crown/roof of the glass tank furnace

2. Coke oven batteries

3. Hot blast stove

TABLE 5.4 Details of the Properties Required for Silica Refractories That Are Used in Different Applications

Properties	Glass Tank Furnace Crown	Coke Oven Batteries	Hot Blast Stove
SiO_2 content (min) %	97	94	94
CaO content (max) %	2	2.5	2.5–3.0
$Al_2O_3 + TiO_2$ content (max) %	0.5	1.5	1.5
Fe_2O_3 content (max) %	0.5	1.5	1.0
Refractoriness, °C	1690	1680	1680
RUL (Ta) °C	1650–1680	1620	1620
Bulk density, g/cc	1.9	1.9	1.8–1.9
Apparent porosity (%)	18–20	18–20	24–26
CCS (Mpa)	35–40	30–35	30–35
Thermal expansion at 1000°C	1.26	1.18–1.2	1.22
PLCR, at 1450°C for 2 h, % (max)	+1.0	+0.4	+0.4
Main phase content	Cristobalite	Tridymite	Tridymite

5.7.1 Crown or Roof of the Glass Tank Furnace

Among the three major applications of silica refractories, this is the most critical one. Continuous glass manufacturing process involves the glass melting tank furnace and the melting chamber of the furnace has the most important function. The reactions amongst the batch materials occur here with the melting of the glass. Figure 5.4a shows the internal view of a glass tank furnace melting zone with the crown or roof. The roof of this melting chamber (as detailed in Figure 5.4b) reaches about 1600°C and remains at such high temperature during the service life of the glass melting tank. So, the refractories need to be very pure for such applications. Silica is preferred as the cristobalite is a very stable phase at that temperature range and also, if due to any reason there is a chipping of refractory, that will mix up with the glass batch (consisting about 75% of silica) without affecting the chemical composition and other properties of glass much.

But this application demands some special requirement of properties in silica refractories. Primarily the refractories have to be very pure (SiO_2 ~96%–97%, CaO ~2.0%–2.5%). Impurities present in the refractory must be very minimum as they affect the performance in the long run at high temperatures and may form liquid phase by reacting with the alkalis (vapor from batch materials) and silica. This may cause dripping of refractory and wear out of the crown. Also, these refractories need to be low in porosity, as porosities may allow the alkali vapor to enter within the refractory and form alkali silicates, which are low melting compounds. The conventional glass is a soda (Na_2O)–lime (CaO)–silica composition and the alkali, that is, Na_2O, fly off with the flame and flue gas, reacts with silica and its mineralizer and impurities, and reduces the liquidus temperature drastically. The liquid phase may even form at a temperature of 800°C in Na_2O–SiO_2 system, thus affecting the roof lining very badly.

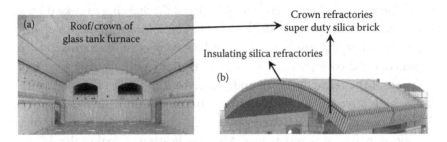

FIGURE 5.4 Roof or crown of the glass melting tank furnace.

The formation of such liquid phases may cause deterioration and collapse of the crown structure. Refractories used in crown need to have high creep resistance as they have to retain the structural integrity at very high temperatures for a prolonged time.

5.7.2 Coke Oven Batteries

Coke is the carbonization product of coal in reducing atmosphere done at about 1100°C after removal of volatile components. Coke is used mainly in the blast furnace for iron making both as a reductant and as a source of thermal energy. At high temperature, it reduces the iron ore and helps to produce liquid metallic iron. Coal is carbonized at high temperature up to a certain degree of volatilization to produce metallurgical coke of desired mechanical and thermochemical properties. Conventional coke making is done in a special type of heat chamber called coke oven and consists of a series of a battery of ovens sandwiched between heating walls. Coal is charged in the coking chamber and it gets heated from the heating chambers on the both sides through the refractory wall. The refractory lining of the coke oven coking chamber at cold condition (open door) is shown in Figure 5.5a and in running condition (closed) as Figure 5.5b, respectively. Figure 5.5c shows the schematic details of the coke oven.

Silica refractory is commonly used in the construction of a coke oven battery. The main reason for selecting silica as a refractory for the coke oven batteries is the very stable tridymite phase of silica refractory in the operating temperature range, which varies between 800°C and 1300°C and a very minimal creep rate at that temperatures. Also, tridymite has the minimum thermal expansion properties among the different crystallographic forms of silica (Figure 5.2), so results in better thermal shock resistance during application. Almost all the expansions of silica brick take place below the coke oven operating temperatures. So during normal operation of the coke oven, fluctuations in temperature due to the opening of the battery during charging of coal and discharging of coke do not affect much on the volume stability of the refractory wall. Again charging and discharging involve friction and abrasion of hard, angular, sharp edged coal and coke particles with the refractory wall, causing wear and abrasion of the refractory wall and the floor. Hence high abrasion resistance, high strength, and low porosity are required for the refractories. The addition of zircon is done to coke oven silica refractories to improve the abrasion and wear resistances. Also, the heating of coal in the coking chamber is done by passing heat through the wall of the heating chambers

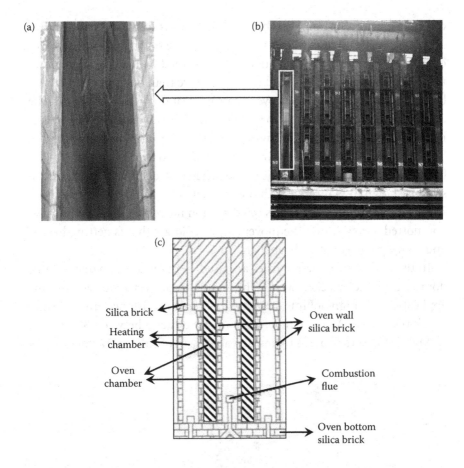

FIGURE 5.5   Coke oven batteries for iron and steel industries.

placed on both the sides. Hence high thermal conductivity with excellent creep resistance at the operating temperatures is required for the refractories. The addition of silicon carbide is also done to improve the thermal conductivity of the refractories. There are many critical shapes and sizes of silica refractories required for coke oven applications, and these are prepared by hand molding techniques. These refractories also need to satisfy the properties as mentioned.

5.7.3 Hot Blast Stove

It is a unit used by the metallurgical industries, especially for iron making, which preheats the air blown into the blast furnace by utilizing the waste heat of the hot flue gases. The stove is a tall, cylindrical steel shell covered unit lined with a refractory. The inner portion is separated into two chambers: a combustion chamber, in which gases from the blast furnace and other fuel sources such as the coke ovens are burnt in the presence of combustion air, and a regenerative chamber lined with a checker work of refractory bricks heated by the burnt gas. More than one stove is required by the industries; when one stove is getting heated by the hot flue gas, the cold air blast passes through the other stove (already preheated) and gets heated by the heat stored in the regenerative chamber on its way to the blast furnace. In this way, the air is preheated up to a maximum of 1300°C before entering the blast furnace. The schematic details of the hot blast stove is shown in Figure 5.6 with the checker silica refractory in the inset. In the figure, solid arrow marks the direction movement of hot waste gas, and dotted arrow shows the movement of cold air that is getting heated and coming out as hot preheated air.

In the stoves, silica refractories are used in many areas, namely walls, domes, and the checker work. The main properties required for this application are high volume stability, high creep resistance, and thermal shock resistance. As the temperature of stove varies between 800°C and 1300°C, tridymite phase is the most stable form of silica refractory, which

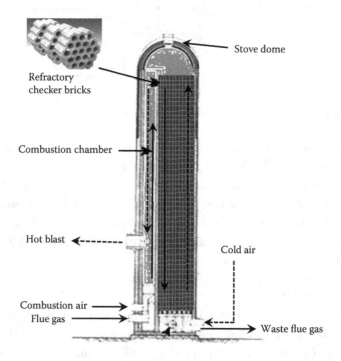

FIGURE 5.6 Schematic of hot blast stove and silica bricks/shapes (inset).

is volumetrically stable and has high creep resistance. Also, high thermal conductivity with low residual quartz content (<1%) and low expansion properties are desirable for this application.

5.8 SILICOSIS

It is also important to know about any harmful effect of the refractories to our biological system. Working for a long time in silica plants where a human is frequently exposed to high silica containing dust, whether produced by cutting and grinding of silica refractory or by quartzite fines, is highly dangerous as it may cause silicosis. As per medical terminology, silicosis is the fibrosis (swelling) of lungs due to inhalation of dust containing silica. Initially, it was believed that silicosis is a purely physical activity where the lungs are lacerated by the sharp and tiny hard grains of silica. Later, it was proved that not only physical but also chemical activity is involved in the disease.

Silicosis occurs due to deposition of fine respirable dust (less than 10 microns in diameter) containing crystalline silica in the form of alpha-quartz, cristobalite, or tridymite. It is characterized by shortness of breath, cough, fever, and cyanosis (bluish skin). It may often be misdiagnosed as pulmonary edema (fluid in the lungs), pneumonia, or tuberculosis.

5.9 SUMMARY

Silica is one of the most abundant minerals available in nature in a pure form and is used for making silica refractory.

Silica has three polymorphic forms, namely quartz, tridymite, and cristobalite, and each form has a low- and high-temperature variations. Each polymorphic form and their temperature-dependent variations transform from one form to another with changing temperature but is associated with volume change. These changes are crucial for silica manufacturing and their applications, as these may result in cracking of the refractory.

Polymorphic transformations are sluggish in nature, and they are not completed during firing. To accelerate them, special chemicals, called mineralizers, are added in silica refractory batch during mixing. To accelerate and stabilize the cristobalite and tridymite phases, CaO and mix of CaO + Fe_2O_3 are added, respectively.

The firing of silica refractories needs to be very slow to accommodate the volume changes without structural disturbances and to crack. The final temperature is dependent on the desired phase in the fired refractory.

The presence of free quartz in fire refractories called residual quartz (RQ) is highly detrimental as it converts to high-temperature forms during firing and use, causing volume expansion, cracks and failure of the refractory.

The properties of the silica refractories are dependent on the purity and amount and types of impurities present. In general, the silica refractory has an RUL value very close to its refractoriness, due to its purity and in case any liquid phase is formed from impurities, the viscosity of the liquid remains very high due to high silica content and deformation of the shape is very less.

Silica refractories are mostly applied to the crown of glass melting tank furnace, coke oven batteries, and hot blast stoves in iron and steel industries.

QUESTIONS AND ASSIGNMENTS

1. Discuss the different crystallographic forms of silica.

2. Why a manufacturer or a user of silica refractory needs to be careful during heating or cooling of the refractory.

3. Describe in detail about the manufacturing technique of silica refractory.

4. Write the precautions during firing of silica refractory.

5. What is a mineralizer? What mineralizers are used in silica refractory?

6. What is Dale's theory or how CaO works in stabilizing silica refractory?

7. Why do silica refractories have RUL values very close to that of refractoriness?

8. Describe the effect of impurities present in silica refractories using the phase diagrams.

9. Describe different applications of silica refractory.

10. Discuss the specific properties required for silica refractories in each of the three main applications.

11. What is residual quartz in silica refractories and how is it important?

12. Why is alumina a harmful impurity in silica refractories?

13. What do you know about silicosis?

BIBLIOGRAPHY

1. J. H. Chesters, *Refractories—Production and Properties*, Woodhead Publishing Ltd., Cambridge, UK, 2006.
2. C. A. Schacht, *Refractories Handbook*, CRC Press, Boca Raton, FL, 2004.
3. P. P. Budnikov, *The Technology of Ceramics and Refractories*, Translated by E. Arnold, *Scripta Technica*, The MIT Press, Cambridge, MA, 4th edn., 2003.
4. A. R. Chesti, *Refractories: Manufacture, Properties and Applications*, Prentice-Hall of India, New Delhi, 1986.
5. *Refractories Handbook*, The Technical Association of Refractories, Japan, 1998.
6. *Harbison-Walker Handbook of Refractory Practice*, Harbison-Walker, PA, 2005.
7. F. Brunk, Silica refractories, *CN Refractories*, Special Issue, 5, 27–30, 2001.
8. F. Brunk, Silica bricks for modern coke oven batteries. *Coke Making International*, 2, 37–40, 2000.
9. I. A. Aksay and J. A. Pask, Stable and metastable equilibria in the system SiO_2-Al_2O_3, *Journal of the American Ceramic Society*, 58(11–12), 507–512, 1975.
10. J. R. Taylor and A. T. Dinsdale, Thermodynamic and phase diagram data for the CaO–SiO_2 system, *Calphad*, 14(1), 71–88, 1990.
11. P. Wu, G. Eriksson, A. D. Pelton, and M. Blander, Prediction of the thermodynamic properties and phase diagrams of silicate systems—Evaluation of FeO–MgO–SiO_2 system, *ISIJ International*, 33(1), 26–35, 1993.
12. R. C. DeVries, R. Roy, and E. F. Osborn, The system TiO_2-SiO_2, *Transactions of the British Ceramic Society*, 53(9), 525–540, 1954.

CHAPTER 6

Alumina Refractories

6.1 INTRODUCTION

Alumina (Al_2O_3) refractories cover a wide range of refractories having a major portion of the total refractory. Any refractory containing more than 50 wt% Al_2O_3 is termed as an alumina refractory. Low alumina-containing (say 50%) refractories are a better version of fireclay refractories having greater volume stability, higher strength both at ambient and elevated temperatures, improved resistances against corrosive attack and better resistances against abrasion and erosion, thermal shock, and creep. The higher amount of Al_2O_3-containing refractories show significantly different and improved properties than those of the low Al_2O_3-containing ones.

During the first half of 1940s, a major development of the Al_2O_3 refractories took place when the use of Al_2O_3–SiO_2 bricks using bauxite as major raw material began in many of the industrial applications. Again the commercial success of the Bayer process for manufacturing very pure alumina (and aluminum) opened up a new horizon for the manufacturing of highly pure alumina refractories. This process also gave an entirely new class of alumina raw materials like calcined and tabular alumina—generating a new line of high Al_2O_3 refractories. Also the parallel development in processing technology like grinding, separation, mixing, pressing, and firing improved dramatically and resulted in a technological edge in the refractory manufacturing. Technical improvements in all types of refractory products caused a reduction in refractory consumption rates. The result has been observed as a decline in production of fireclay-based Al_2O_3–SiO_2 refractories.

Alumina refractories have silica as the second most prominent oxide phase, and they cover the major portion of the Al_2O_3–SiO_2 phase equilibrium diagram, as shown in Figure 6.1. Low alumina and high silica-containing regions of the phase diagram represent the silica and fireclay refractories. If we increase the alumina content in pure silica composition (starting from zero level), the refractories that appear first are super-duty silica refractory (~97% SiO_2 and ~0.5% Al_2O_3). A little increase in alumina content and reduction in silica produces the general-purpose silica refractory (~94% SiO_2 and ~2% Al_2O_3). An increase in alumina produces the semisilica fireclay refractory

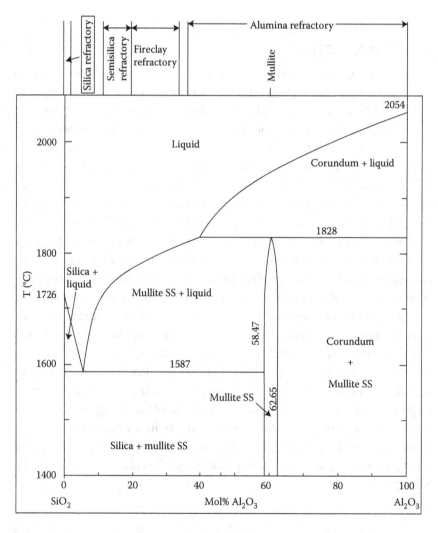

FIGURE 6.1   Phase diagram of alumina–silica system.

(65%–80% SiO_2 and 18%–25% Al_2O_3). A further increase in alumina content produces the fireclay refractories, containing approximately 25–45 wt% Al_2O_3, and then comes the alumina refractories. Again the alumina refractories are classified according to their Al_2O_3 content. Generally the classifications are 50%, 60%, 70%, 80%, 90%, and 99% Al_2O_3-containing refractories. All the major classes of refractories based on the Al_2O_3–SiO_2 phase diagram are shown in Figure 6.1 for better understanding.

It can be seen from the phase diagram that the refractoriness of the refractory increases with the increase in the Al_2O_3 content. The only eutectic present is at 1587°C has a composition of 94.5% SiO_2 and 5.5% Al_2O_3 and is far away from the alumina refractories. The only compound, mullite ($3Al_2O_3$ $2SiO_2$), forms at a composition of 71.8 wt% Al_2O_3 and 28.2 wt% SiO_2. There are different opinions regarding the melting behavior of mullite; according to a group of researchers, it is a congruent melting compound having a sharp melting point at 1840°C and, in contradiction, some researchers found it as an incongruently melting compound with decomposition and liquid formation at 1828°C. As on today, mullite is being considered as an incongruently melting compound with a defective lattice structure that allows formation of solid solution on both the sides of the composition, as described by Aksay and Pask and Figure 6.1 represents their work.

6.2 RAW MATERIALS AND SOURCES

Aluminum is the third most abundant element in the earth's crust, and so plenty of aluminum-bearing minerals are available in nature. But nearly no naturally occurring commercial source is available in the pure oxide form. Most commonly available minerals containing a high amount of alumina with minimum impurities are used as raw materials for alumina refractories. As the alumina content varies widely in alumina refractories (say from 50% to 99%), different types of natural (few synthetic) raw materials are used, having different amounts alumina, to obtain the required alumina content in the final composition economically. Synthetic raw materials are used for making very high pure alumina refractories, whose purity level is difficult to obtain from natural sources and also to impart some special properties in the refractories. The commonly used raw materials for alumina are as follows.

6.2.1 Fireclay

Details of the fireclay are described in Chapter 7, dealing with fireclay refractories. For making alumina refractories with low alumina content

(50%–60% Al_2O_3), calcined fireclays are used in combination with some high alumina clays (commonly termed as diasporic clay or bauxitic clays) or natural aluminosilicate minerals. A good quality calcined fireclay contains 40%–45% Al_2O_3 and to get the balanced amount of alumina the batch composition is adjusted with the higher alumina-containing raw materials.

6.2.2 Anhydrous Aluminosilicates

Naturally occurring anhydrous aluminosilicates, namely sillimanite, kyanite, and andalusite, are having the same chemical formula, Al_2SiO_5, but different crystal structures. These differences in crystal structure give somewhat unique physical properties to each of the three minerals, and each one is used in slightly different ways. In theoretically pure form, the aluminosilicates contain 62.9% Al_2O_3 and 37.1% SiO_2 but the natural resources are impure, and alumina content is less than 60%. The main impurities present are Fe_2O_3, TiO_2, and CaO. Sillimanite is not widely available and used in lesser extent due to limited availability in rock form. Some beach sand sources of sillimanite are available in a very few countries. Comparatively, much greater availability and widely used mineral is kyanite. Kyanite is also sometimes mixed with quartz as impurity. Andalusite is also widely available throughout the globe, but many sources are associated with pyrophyllitic clay as an impurity.

These aluminosilicate compounds are not present in the very common Al_2O_3–SiO_2 phase diagram that shows the equilibrium at 1 atm pressure. None of these three minerals are equilibrium phases at 1 atm. These are formed at higher-pressure and higher-temperature geological conditions and all are available as a metastable phase in nature. On heating, these metastable aluminosilicates convert to equilibrium stable mullite phase and free silica glass. The temperature of this decomposition and mullite formation changes from one mineral to another. Table 6.1 summarizes the properties of these three natural aluminosilicates and the differences among them.

6.2.3 Bauxite

Bauxite is the principal aluminum ore and consists mostly of the minerals gibbsite [$Al(OH)_3$], boehmite [γ-$AlO(OH)$], and diaspore [α-$AlO(OH)$]. Truly speaking, bauxite is not a mineral, but rather a group of aluminum hydroxides. The term is used to describe the economically important mixture of these minerals, which form a mass of the individually classified members of gibbsite, boehmite, and diaspore. All the bauxites that are

TABLE 6.1 Properties of Sillimanite, Kyanite, and Andalusite

	Sillimanite	Kyanite	Andalusite
Crystal system	Orthorhombic	Triclinic	Orthorhombic
Specific gravity	3.23	3.56–3.66	3.16–3.20
Hardness, Mohs scale	6–7	5–7	7.5
Mullite formation temperature	1550–1650°C	1100–1480°C	1450–1500°C
Volume changes on calcination	Slight increase	Very large increase	Very slight increase
Specific gravity after calcination	3.10	3.05	3.04
Fusion temperature	>1800°C	>1800°C	>1800°C

available in nature are not easily extractable, and separation of the aluminum-bearing mineral is sometimes difficult or a costly affair. The bauxites that involve a less complicated process to get aluminum-containing phases are called as recoverable bauxites and those sources and reserves are economically important. Again the major application of bauxite is for manufacturing of aluminum metal that involves a chemical treatment of raw bauxite first to separate out the only aluminum phase. Thus, purity of this metallurgical grade bauxite may be little compromised as chemical reactions involved in the processing to separate out the impurities from the system easily. But for use in refractory industries, the bauxite is only calcined without any chemical treatment. Hence, the refractory grade bauxites need to purer.

Ideally, bauxite should contain 73.9% Al_2O_3 and 26.1% H_2O and on the calcined basis, it is 100% Al_2O_3. In natural occurrence, mixtures of gibbsite and boehmite are common in bauxite and mix of boehmite and diaspore is less common and gibbsite and diaspore are rare. Some high-grade refractory bauxite consists solely of gibbsite with minor amounts of kaolin clay [$Al_2Si_2O_5(OH)_4$]. The common impurities found in both metallurgical and refractory grade bauxites are aluminosilicate (mainly clay), quartz (SiO_2), hematite (Fe_2O_3), goethite [$FeO(OH)$], rutile (TiO_2), and anatase (TiO_2). Hematite and goethite are the most abundant iron impurities in many bauxites and the principal reason for the red and brown colors that are characteristic of countless bauxite deposits.

The world's bauxite resources are estimated to be 55–75 billion tons. But all the reserve is not viable for commercial exploitation and the recoverable reserves are estimated to be around 25 billion tons. The largest recoverable reserves are in Australia followed by Guinea, Brazil, Jamaica, and India. Among different non-metallurgical grades of bauxite, the refractory grade is the purest one. A bauxite to be used in refractories should have at least 58% of Al_2O_3 content, and the impurities that may be allowed are a max of 5% of SiO_2, ~3% of TiO_2 max and 3% of Fe_2O_3. Since bauxites give away their water during heating accompanied by a marked reduction in volume, they are calcined and sintered before used in refractories. During this sintering, corundum and mullite phases are formed, together with a small amount of low melting liquid phase containing iron and titanium. Despite the presence of low melting phase, bauxite can only be densified to a compact on sintering at high temperatures.

6.2.4 Synthetic Raw Materials

Naturally occurring mineral, mainly bauxite, is purified by chemical treatment to remove the impurities and then calcined produces synthetic alumina. It was initially produced from bauxite in 1888 using the Bayer process. Synthetic alumina is available mainly in three forms: activated alumina, smelter-grade alumina, and calcined alumina. The porous, granular activated alumina aggressively absorbs liquid water and water vapor. Smelter-grade alumina is used for making aluminum metal. The fine-grain calcined alumina is a dense impermeable ceramic material used for abrasives, refractories, electrical insulation, high-temperature crucibles, and dental restoration. It is also used as a filler for paints, glass, and ceramics.

Fused alumina is also used for making alumina refractories mainly to improve the corrosion resistance. It is produced by the electrofusion route. In fused alumina, alumina crystals grow from a molten stage, and the growth rate is very high compared to solid state growth resulting in very large crystals when solidified as fused alumina. Large crystals have lesser numbers of grain and grain boundaries, resulting in lesser surface area for reaction by any corrosive agent, which improves corrosion resistance. Fused alumina can be prepared from the bauxite directly having impurities like iron oxide, silica, and titania with a reddish, yellowish, or brownish color called brown-fused alumina. Again a white-fused alumina with minimum impurities can also be obtained by fusing Bayer's process purer alumina.

Sintered alumina is another variety of synthetic alumina prepared from finely ground calcined Al_2O_3 by sintering it below its melting point. As a result of this high-temperature sintering process, the properties are excellent and, in particular, a uniform crystal structure with high strength both at ambient and elevated temperatures.

There is also a special class of sintered alumina called tabular alumina in which shaping of high pure calcined alumina and its sintering at very high temperature is done in such a way that enables the alpha-alumina crystals to grow into large grains, of a form resembling tablets, hence termed as "tabular" alumina. In this processing, the alumina, which has been shaped into spheres for firing, shrinks and results in a uniform microstructure with low residual porosity. The spheres are mainly crushed and ground into a range of particle size distributions. These aluminas have excellent properties like high density, low open porosity, dimensional stability, creep and abrasion resistance, exceptional resistance to thermal shock, and uniform, compact microstructure.

Synthetic mullite ($Al_6Si_2O_{13}$) is also used as a raw material for some special alumina refractories, produced by the sintering process or fusion. In the process, the initial materials clay or kaolin are enriched in alumina content to have a composition of mullite by the addition of calcined Al_2O_3. The mixture is then electrofused or pressed and sintered as specified in processing, and the fired products are crushed and ground to get the desired particle fractions.

6.3 A BRIEF OF MANUFACTURING TECHNIQUES

Alumina refractories cover a wide class of refractories having a wide variety of alumina content and other secondary oxides. Accordingly, the raw materials also vary according to the composition of the refractory to optimize the properties and economy. Table 6.2 shows of the classification of refractories under this broad class of alumina refractory and the main raw materials used for making them.

Alumina refractories are manufactured by the typical manufacturing process of refractory making. Different fractions of the raw materials are taken and mixed in pan, muller, and countercurrent mixer initially as dried condition, and then green binders, and moisture are added for

TABLE 6.2 Raw Materials Combination for Different Alumina Refractories

Refractory Class	Raw Materials Used
50% Al_2O_3	Fireclay, diasporic clay, aluminosilicates, bauxite
60% Al_2O_3	Aluminosilicate, bauxite, fireclay, bauxite clay
70% Al_2O_3	Bauxite, aluminosilicates, bauxite clay
80% Al_2O_3	Bauxite
90% Al_2O_3	Bauxite, synthetic alumina
>95% Al_2O_3	Synthetic alumina

proper binding and handling strength at the green and dried conditions. Mixed batch is then shaped by pressing and then dried and fired. Pressing of alumina refractories is done in mechanical, friction screw, or hydraulic presses. Binders and moisture also impart some plastic character to the mix to retain the shape after pressing and shaping. Firing is done in both batch, or continuous type of kilns and the temperature is dependent on the composition, especially on the alumina content. Firing temperature may vary from 1450°C to 1750°C.

6.4 CLASSIFICATIONS AND PROPERTIES

The classification of alumina refractories is done as per the alumina content, and obviously the properties will also vary. Table 6.3 shows a general idea about the properties of the different alumina refractories including a general chemical composition of each category. In general, the second component in the alumina refractories is silica, which reacts with alumina and forms mullite. Mullite, having a high volume stability, lower thermal expansion, high creep resistance, and high thermal shock resistance, is beneficial for alumina refractories. But the presence of impurities like iron oxide, titania, lime, and alkalis may react with alumina and alumiosilicate phases and form low-melting compounds, thus strongly deteriorating the high-temperature properties. An increasing amount of alumina content produces a better refractory with higher strength, density, and heat properties. The presence of higher amount of iron oxide may reduce the thermo-mechanical properties (say, RUL) drastically even the composition may have a higher alumina content. Also, at high temperatures, alumina shows a little acidic character and may form compounds on reaction with highly basic materials.

TABLE 6.3 Properties of Different Alumina Refractories

Refractory Class	Al_2O_3 (%)	Fe_2O_3 (%)	BD (g/cc)	AP (%)	CCS (MPa)	RUL, Ta (°C)
50% Al_2O_3	50	1.3	2.35	18	35	1500
60% Al_2O_3	60	3	2.4	22	40	1450
62% Al_2O_3	62	1.2	2.5	16	60	1550
70% Al_2O_3	70	2.5	2.6	20	40	1480
70% Al_2O_3 (mullite)	70	0.8	2.55	18	60	1680
80% Al_2O_3	80	2.5	2.7	22	50	1500
85% Al_2O_3	85	1.5	2.9	18	60	1600
90% Al_2O_3	88 min	0.5	2.95	18	65	1700
95% Al_2O_3	94 min	0.5	3.0	22	70	1700
99% Al_2O_3	97 min	0.1	~3.1	18	75	1750

However, as the same quality of alumina refractory can be prepared by a different source of raw materials, so the properties may again vary as per the raw materials used. Accordingly the applications are to be selected. Otherwise, the same amount of alumina containing refractory may perform differently. For example, 50% and 60% Al_2O_3 containing refractory, when prepared from bauxite or andalusite, typically exhibit high reheat expansion while refractories based on clay (fireclay, diasporic/bauxite clay) do not. Thus, there is a fundamental difference in the refractories within the same class (same Al_2O_3%) on permanent expansion characteristics. In linings requiring the extreme tightness (as in rotary kiln applications), the reheat expansion is extremely important and improves the lining life. But in contrast, high reheat expansion may be associated with the high spalling tendency, that is, low spalling resistance. In this regard, refractories produced from a clay base material have superior properties. This is because of their finer texture, smaller average pore size, and due to the absence of permanent expansion on heating. A similar kind of character is also evident for the 70% Al_2O_3-containing refractories.

The presence of higher amount of impurities, say iron oxide content, will reduce the liquidus temperature by forming low melting compounds on reaction with alumina and silica present and will result in lower hot strength (RUL) properties. Thus, the same class of refractory may have different properties and will have different applications.

Refractories containing Al_2O_3 in the range of 80%–85% were originally developed for use in aluminum smelting and holding furnaces. These refractories are purely based on calcined bauxite, as it is the closest mineral in Al_2O_3 content to their overall composition. The resistance against molten aluminum and salt fluxes for these refractories arises from the resistance of the bauxite. But these refractories are not highly successful in the ferrous industry. The reason for that is the processing temperature. The aluminum industry operates at a much lower temperature than the ferrous industries and at higher temperatures, the bond phase (glass and mullite) of the refractories, holding together highly refractory calcined bauxite aggregate particles, gets softened. Hence in an aggressive slagging situation, the bauxite aggregate is eroded out of the refractory brick due to weak and viscous bond phase and the wear rates are unusually high.

Refractories containing Al_2O_3 in the range of 90% or above are having the highest strength and erosion and corrosion resistance and heat properties. They are made from synthetic Al_2O_3 aggregates, and some types may contain fused Al_2O_3 for special corrosion and erosion resistance.

Depending upon the impurity phase and its quantity the bond phase may be mullite-based or alumina-based ones. Alumina-bonded alumina refractories (direct bond) results in superior properties, especially the corrosion and heat strength properties.

There is a practical limit on Al_2O_3 content in high-alumina refractories [~96% Al_2O_3 (contains ~3% SiO_2)] for very high temperature applications. Products containing further higher Al_2O_3 content are difficult to sinter in conventional firing techniques and industrially available temperatures (~1750°C). These refractories show comparatively poor properties especially from density, strength, and reheat change (PLCR) points of view. Though 99% Al_2O_3-containing refractories exist, they are primarily used for low-temperature applications, mainly for their inertness (chemical resistance).

6.5 EFFECT OF IMPURITIES ON PHASE DIAGRAMS

Impurities are also very effective in affecting the properties of the alumina refractories. The most common impurities present with alumina are mainly silica, iron oxide, titania, and alkalis. In most of the alumina refractories, silica is the second major component and presence of only silica does not deteriorate the properties of alumina very strongly. As seen in Figure 6.1, the presence of silica in alumina will produce a mixture of corundum and mullite solid solution, and a liquid phase appears at 1828°C and above which the phase composition changes to corundum and liquid. The composition and amount of the liquid changes with the amount of silica present in the system and the temperature. Hence the presence of only silica as impurity will reduce the liquid formation temperature up to 1828°C, which is above the general application temperature of the alumina refractories and so deterioration in high-temperature properties does not affect the performance.

The presence of iron oxide also affects the liquidus and reduces the liquid formation temperature, but the effect is also not so pronounced. For Fe_2O_3, alumina forms a corundum solid solution at high temperature, thus absorbing the ferric ions in the corundum structure and so the properties are hardly affected, as shown in Figure 6.2a. Again at a higher level of Fe_2O_3, the liquid phase starts forming from 1689°C and a mixture of corundum solid solution with liquid phase was obtained above this temperature. For FeO, the liquid phase starts forming at 1750°C, which is the eutectic temperature in the system. Also a congruent melting spinel compound forms in the system, named hercynite ($FeAl_2O_4$, containing about

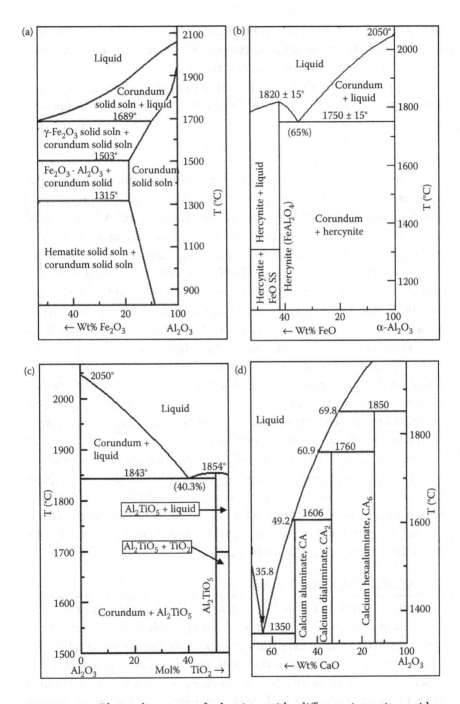

FIGURE 6.2 Phase diagrams of alumina with different impurity oxides: (a) Fe_2O_3, (b) FeO, (c) TiO_2, and (d) CaO.

58% Al_2O_3) with a melting point of 1820°C. Hence presence of only iron oxide as an impurity in alumina system, as a ferric or ferrous state, does not affect the high temperature properties strongly.

The presence of titania also showed similar characteristics as that of FeO, forming a eutectic and also forms a congruent melting compound, aluminum titanate. Eutectic is at 1843°C and the compound melts at 1854°C. Hence, only TiO_2 is also not very effective in deteriorating the properties of alumina. But the presence of lime (CaO) in alumina is effective in reducing the liquidus temperature. The temperature decreases with the increasing amount of lime content and a number of incongruent melting compounds also form in the system. The alumina-rich compound is calcium hexaaluminate (CA_6), which incongruently melts at 1850°C. A further increase in CaO produces calcium dialuminate (CA_2), which decomposes to liquid and CA_6 at 1760°C. On further increase in CaO, calcium aluminate is formed, which incongruently melts to CA_2 and liquid at 1606°C. The lowest temperature of liquid formation in the $CaO-Al_2O_3$ system is at 1350°C, which is a eutectic of the system, having only about 36% alumina content. Though this composition is never reached in alumina refractories, but at the zonal presence of CaO, there may be an initiation of the liquid phase at the proximity of the lime particles present. Hence, that may affect the whole system. This temperature is quite low compared to any refractory application temperatures and so the presence of lime in alumina needs to be carefully checked.

However, in actual case, none of the impurities are present singly in the alumina system, and so compound effect of all the different impurities exist, which is much stronger and effective in deteriorating the high-temperature properties of alumina. Understanding of such type of effects necessarily requires the study of multicomponent systems and presently kept outside of the scope of this book.

6.6 MAIN APPLICATION AREAS

Alumina is a commonly available material and has excellent chemical, thermal, and mechanical properties both at ambient and elevated temperatures. Due to these excellent refractory qualities, alumina refractory is very common. For most of the application areas of refractories, if the specific required refractory is not available, one can use high alumina refractory and can run the high-temperature process. But the presence of impurities in the refractory and the environment, as described, restricts its use. Table 6.4 presents details about the different application areas of

TABLE 6.4   Applications of Different Alumina-Containing Refractories

Refractory Class	Application Area
50% Al_2O_3	Preheater of cement rotary kiln; anode baking furnace; glass tank regenerators.
	They are mainly used as an upgraded version of fireclay refractories. They have relatively low porosities and expansive nature up to about 1600°C, minimizing the joint gap between the bricks, resulting in a compact lining. These refractories have low thermal expansion and good spalling resistances and are the preferred choice for backup lining for many high-temperature industries. As the major second phase is silica, with less harmful impurities, these refractories are an excellent choice for preheaters and calcining zones of the rotary kilns.
60% Al_2O_3	Blast furnace stove checkers; blast furnace lining, preheating zones of cement rotary kilns.
	Refractories produced from calcined bauxitic clay and high-purity kaolin have a lower level of harmful impurities, resulting in low porosity, high heat strength, and creep resistance with excellent volume stability at high temperatures. The use of bauxite imparts iron oxide as an impurity and deteriorates the high-temperature properties.
62% Al_2O_3	Blast furnace hearth and tuyere; blast furnace stove checker.
	Low impurity and high firing results in excellent load bearing capacity, heat strength, and creep resistance, primarily required for blast furnace hearth applications. Impurities, like iron oxide, must be minimum for hearth applications.
70% Al_2O_3	Electric arc furnace roof; steel ladle, rotary kiln.
	This is the most commonly used high alumina refractory and one of the best refractories for performance to cost ratio. They are prepared mainly from calcined bauxite and high-grade clay. In many cases, the refractories are fired at a lower temperature to have lower expansions, which occur during application at high temperatures due to the reaction between alumina sources with silica available in the composition forming low-dense mullite phase associated with expansion. This secondary expansion during application is beneficial to reduce the joint size and gap between the bricks, resulting in a tight and compact refractory lining, highly useful for the rotary kiln, and steel ladle applications.
70% Al_2O_3 (mullite) (low iron)	Blast furnace hearth and tap hole; glass tank furnace.
	Special attention is given to the formation of mullite in the composition. High temperature and prolong firing is used with reduced impurity level to complete the mullitization reaction and maximize the mullite crystal development. Excellent resistances against silicate liquids with high heat strength and creep resistances are the most important character of mullite-based refractory, which is essentially utilized in the blast furnace and glass tank furnace applications.

(Continued)

TABLE 6.4 (*Continued*) Applications of Different Alumina-Containing Refractories

Refractory Class	Application Area
80%–85% Al_2O_3	Electric arc furnace roof, steel ladle, aluminum melting and holding furnace; torpedo ladle.
	These refractories are mostly based on bauxite only and in some cases fine high pure clay or aluminas. They are also relatively common and widely used in various industries. They possess good strength and thermal shock resistances and work well against various slag conditions and extensively used in steel and aluminum industries.
90% Al_2O_3	Reheating furnace hearth; carbon black reactor.
	These refractories are mostly based on synthetic alumina, namely tabular and fused alumina grains and technical alumina fines with high pure bauxite fines. They mostly consist of corundum and mullite phase and possess high heat strength and excellent resistances against creep and chemical attack.
95%–99% Al_2O_3	Chemical, petrochemical, and fertilizer industries, ceramic kilns.
	Very high pure alumina refractories are made from synthetic raw materials and possess only corundum as a constituting phase. Extreme high purity may require a very high temperature of firing, which sometimes is not practically feasible, resulting in relatively lower densification and strength properties as that is expected. The applications of these refractories in corrosive atmosphere of different chemical industries are mainly due to their excellent corrosion resistances coming from their purity. Use in high-temperature ceramic kilns is also important for their high-temperature withstanding capacity.

different subclasses of alumina refractories. Obviously low-alumina-containing refractories are marginally better than fireclay refractories and used in low-temperature applications, whereas application temperature and criticality of the application increase with increasing amount of alumina content. Again refractories containing >97% alumina are difficult to sinter in bulk shape under industrial and commercial conditions and so fired products have relatively poor qualities compared to their alumina content and as expected. Hence, these refractories are used mostly as a pure refractory material with high chemical resistances, and not for high-temperature properties. Some of the application areas of different types of alumina refractories are shown in Figure 6.3.

6.7 SUMMARY

Alumina is the only compound formed between aluminum and oxygen, the third and first most abundant elements in the earth's crust. Hence, it is abundantly available in nature but not available as oxide form.

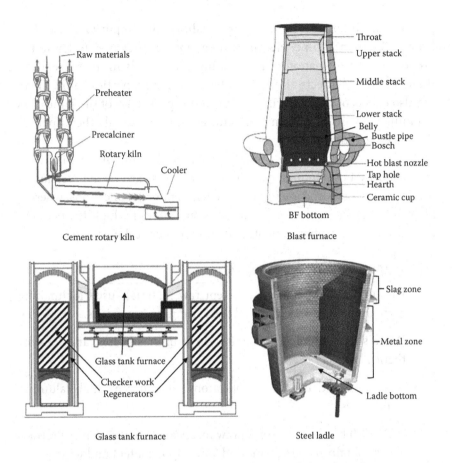

Cement rotary kiln

Blast furnace

Glass tank furnace

Steel ladle

FIGURE 6.3 Some application areas and industries of alumina refractories.

The main raw material sources for alumina refractories are fireclay and all other high alumina clays, like diasporic clay, bauxitic clay, etc; natural aluminosilicates, namely, sillimanite, kyanite, and andalusite; bauxite and synthetic alumina like fused alumina, tabular alumina, calcined and sintered alumina, and synthetic mullite. These raw materials mostly in combination with one another are used to make alumina refractories of different alumina contents.

The conventional refractory manufacturing technique of mixing, pressing, and firing is used to make the refractory shapes. Firing temperature varies with alumina content and for very high pure refractories, it is about 1750°C.

All the properties of the alumina refractories vary with purity. The main secondary phase present is silica, which forms mullite in the fired product and improves the refractory qualities. But impurity phases like iron oxide, titania, lime, etc. in combination drastically deteriorate the properties. The formation of low melting compounds in the presence of these impurities affects all the high-temperature properties badly. There are also effects of raw material sources on the properties of the same class (alumina content) of alumina refractories and accordingly their applications need to judge.

Alumina refractories are applied in vivid areas with wide variation in temperatures. Low alumina containing refractories are a better version of fireclay refractories and are used in low-temperature applications, whereas high alumina containing compositions are used in high-temperature critical application environments and also for chemical inertness.

QUESTIONS AND ASSIGNMENTS

1. Discuss briefly about the different raw materials used for making high alumina refractories and their common impurities.

2. Write short note on (a) bauxite, (b) aluminosilicates, and (c) synthetic alumina.

3. Describe in detail the applications of different high alumina refractories.

4. What will be the variation in raw materials to make alumina refractories containing 50%, 80%, and 90% Al_2O_3 content and why?

5. Describe the complete manufacturing method of a high-alumina refractory.

6. What are the advantages of having mullite phase in high-alumina refractories?

7. Draw the Al_2O_3–SiO_2 phase diagram, describe the same, and indicate in the diagram different refractory systems that are based on this phase diagram.

8. What are the major impurity phases present in alumina refractories and discuss their effects on the properties?

9. Why silica alone is not highly detrimental in alumina refractories? Discuss with a phase diagram.

10. Why do higher alumina containing refractories show lower RUL values in some cases?

11. Discuss why the same class of alumina refractory based on aluminosilicates are good for cement rotary kilns but not good for steel ladle.

BIBLIOGRAPHY

1. J. H. Chesters, *Refractories—Production and Properties*, Woodhead Publishing Ltd., Cambridge, UK, 2006.
2. C. A. Schacht, *Refractories Handbook*, CRC Press, Boca Raton, FL, 2004.
3. P. P. Budnikov, *The Technology of Ceramics and Refractories*, 4th edn., translated by E. Arnold, *Scripta Technica*, The MIT Press, Cambridge, MA, 2003.
4. A. R. Chesti, *Refractories: Manufacture, Properties and Applications*, Prentice-Hall of India, New Delhi, 1986.
5. *Refractories Handbook*, The Technical Association of Refractories, Japan, 1998.
6. *Harbison-Walker Handbook of Refractory Practice*, Harbison-Walker, PA, 2005.
7. A. O. Surendranathan, *An Introduction to Ceramics and Refractories*, CRC Press, Boca Raton, FL, 2014.
8. *Bauxite, Indian Minerals Yearbook 2013 (Part-III: Mineral Reviews)*, 52nd edn., Indian Bureau of Mines, Ministry of Mines, Govt. of India, January 2015.
9. P. C. Sweet, G. B. Dixon, and J. R. Snoddy, Kyanite, andalusite, sillimanite, and mullite, in *Industrial Minerals & Rocks: Commodities, Markets, and Uses*, J. E. Kogel, N. C. Trivedi (eds.), James M. Barker and Stanley T. Krukowsk, Society for Mining, Metallurgy and Exploration Inc., Englewood, CO, pp. 553–560, 2006.
10. Vincent G. Hill and Errol D. Sehnke, Bauxite, in *Industrial Minerals & Rocks: Commodities, Markets, and Uses*, J. E. Kogel, N. C. Trivedi (eds.), James M. Barker and Stanley T. Krukowsk, Society for Mining, Metallurgy and Exploration Inc., Englewood, CO, pp. 227–261, 2006.
11. I. A. Aksay and J. A. Pask, Stable and metastable equilibria in the system SiO_2–Al_2O_3, *Journal of the American Ceramic Society*, 58(11–12), 507–512, 1975.
12. I. A. Novokhatskii, B. F. Belov, A. V. Gorokh, and A. A. Savinskaya, The phase diagram for the system ferrous oxide-alumina, *Russian Journal of Physics and Chemistry*, 39(11), 1498–1499, 1965.
13. T. I. Barry, A. T. Dinsdale, J. A. Gisby, B. Hallstedt, M. Hillert, S. Jonsson, B. Sundman, and J. R. Taylor, The compound energy model for ionic solutions with applications to solid oxides, *Journal of Phase Equilibria*, 13(5), 459–475, 1992.

14. M. Kirschen, C. DeCapitani, F. Millot, J. C. Rifflet, and J. P. Coutures, Immiscible silicate liquids in the system SiO_2–TiO_2–Al_2O_3, *European Journal of Mineralogy*, 11(3), 427–440, 1999.

15. A. I. Zaitsev, N. V. Korolev, and B. M. Mogutnov, Phase equilibria in the CaF_2–Al_2O_3–CaO system, *Journal of Material Sciences*, 26(6), 1588–1600, 1991.

CHAPTER 7

Fireclay Refractories

7.1 INTRODUCTION

Fireclay refractories (also commonly known as firebrick) are the most common refractories and important types from the view of total volume production. They are based on clay and hydrated aluminosilicate and contain silica and alumina as the main constituents and so often comes under a broad class of aluminosilicate refractories. In general, fireclay refractories contain about 25–45 wt% of alumina and the major component of the rest is silica. These refractories are one of the oldest ones that was started to protect heat and run a high-temperature process. But, as the knowledge increases, newer refractories have come up with appropriate and specific properties suitable for certain specific applications and slowly the use of fireclay refractories is discarded. But it is one of the most common refractories that is used for low-temperature applications and as the backup lining of many high-temperature processes. When comparing with other refractories, fireclay refractories are inferior to silica and basic refractories in resistance to chemical attack against acidic and basic environments, respectively and weaker both at ambient and elevated temperatures to alumina refractories.

Fireclay is a hydrated aluminosilicate, and so the refractory is based on the alumina–silica phase diagram, as detailed in the previous chapter (Figure 6.1). The portion of the phase diagram having alumina content between 25 and 45 wt% of alumina represents the portion of fireclay refractories. As per the phase diagram, the lowest temperature of liquid formation for pure fireclay is at 1587°C, the eutectic temperature. However, presence of impurities strongly affects the high-temperature properties of the fireclay refractories, and the lowering of liquid formation temperature depends on the type and amount of the impurities. The effect of different impurity oxides individually on silica and alumina are shown in Figures 5.2 and 6.2, respectively.

7.2 RAW MATERIALS AND SOURCES

Fireclay is a relatively impure secondary clay commonly found from areas close to coal mines, although other natural deposits are also available as potential sources in many countries. Clays found close to coal mines are often partially fired. Volatile matters of coal may come out through the porous earthy materials above the coal belt and catch fire at atmospheric conditions. This fire also burns the clay mass on the surface and the associated region. Hence, the clay mass close to the coal reserves are partially fired and so these clays are termed as "fireclay." There is also another opinion: clays that are resistant to fire is "fireclay." As a refractory, fireclay found use from the very ancient times and even as on today other than the direct high-temperature hot face applications, it is the most common choice, widely used for making chimney and flue liners. Backup lining in most of the high-temperature operations and fire-resistant pads for safety, as seen when a hearth in front of a fireplace, are used to reduce the risk of fire.

As a secondary clay, it is transported from its formation site and acquires impurities mostly during transportation and got finer too. Like other clays, fireclay is malleable (deformable) in raw form (when wet) due to its plasticity. It can be molded, extruded, shaped by hand, and stamped. But its plasticity varies depending on its nature of origin and constituents present. As per mineralogy, it is a form of kaolinite ($Al_2O_3 \, 2SiO_2 \, 2H_2O$) and theoretically contains about 39.5% alumina, 46.5% silica, and 14% water. In a loss-free basis, fireclay contains about 46% alumina and 54% silica. But fireclay is associated with impurities like Fe_2O_3, TiO_2, CaO, etc. Due to partial firing before mining (mainly the sources close to coal mines), the water content is lower in the clay structure and varies from one source to another. Hence, its plasticity is lower compared to another kaolinite type of clays. Due to this lower and non-uniform plasticity, these clays are not useful for conventional ceramic products manufacturing where plasticity of clay is of the prime importance. Also the presence of impurities does not result in a good white color after firing, and fireclay is not well accepted in "whiteware industries." But for refractories, plasticity and color are of less significance. Also, the presence of lesser extent of structural water in fireclay is beneficial as less heat (and fuel) is required to remove the structural water (during calcination) for making the refractory.

When the fireclay is heated up to 500–600°C, kaolin minerals lose their crystallization water and an intermediate phase, known as metakaolin, is formed. However, this phase still exhibits a low crystalline order. The kaolin lattice does not disintegrate completely until about 950°C. Initially, there is no reaction between the silica and alumina of the decomposed clay, but with further heating around 1000°C, mullite begins to form. Above 1100°C, only mullite, cristobalite, and glassy phases are present. The glassy phase is mainly a silica-based composition (~80% silica and only about 10% alumina, and ~5% of alkalis and alkaline earth minerals). The formation and amount of mullite phase developed in the fired products are dependent on the total alumina content of the clay. Hence, the fireclay refractory has some glassy phase in its microstructure with mullite and cristobalite as crystalline phases.

7.3 GROG AND ITS IMPORTANCE

As fireclay is a secondary clay and transported from its origin of formation, by water, air, etc., it gets finer due to abrasion, erosion during transportation, and consists of very fine particles. Hence, use of only raw clay for making the refractory shape will result in huge shrinkage during drying and firing with associated dangers of cracking, warping, and breakage. So, only raw clay is not used for making the refractory and a material with similar composition but having minimum shrinkage is required to be added.

A part of the clay is calcined before use, and the calcined clay is used along with the raw clay to make the final refractory composition. This prefired calcined clay is termed as "grog." Grog acts as an antishrinkage material in the fireclay composition. For better packing and compaction, we need a green mixture of refractory comprising of different fractions of particles, namely, coarse, medium, and fine particles. This grog is crushed and ground to get the desired fractions of the refractory body. Raw clay is used as the finer fraction in the composition. To make the fireclay refractory economic, crushing of already fired broken bricks or scraps (but not contaminated) are also used as grog. Sharp angular grains of grog results in better interlocking in the shaped compositions and results in higher compaction, density, strength, and other associated properties. Grog is a major component in fireclay refractories, but the quantity of grog varies from one product to another and also the properties. Grog content varies in the range of 20%–90% and rest is raw clay. A high percentage of grog requires highly plastic raw clay to develop proper plasticity in the mix and strength at unfired conditions. Lower grog containing refractories have lower density and strength values. Different advantages of using grogs are as follows:

1. Reduction in shrinkage (chances of warpage and cracking) of the brick on firing
2. Higher density and lower porosity due to better packing
3. Increase strength values
4. Less requirement of water for mixing

7.4 MANUFACTURING OF FIRECLAY REFRACTORIES

Mined raw clay is first moistened and kept in an open atmosphere in thin layers for decaying of organic matters present in it. This helps to form some organic acids (humic acid) from the organic masses present in it, which increases the plasticity of clay. This process is called "weathering or souring." Weathered clays are then crushed and ground. Mainly, the raw clay is used as a fine fraction to make use of its plasticity in the refractory composition. This clay is mixed with the grog fractions, as per the total grog content. A blend of two or more clays is normally done for the manufacture of fireclay refractories to accommodate any variation in any of the clays without much variations in processing and the final properties. No separate green binder is required and used as raw clay itself is a plasticizing and bonding material in the green stage.

The mixture of different grog fractions and fine raw clay is mixed both in dry or wet conditions. In dry conditions, the ingredients are directly charged in the mixer (generally pan mixer) and mixed with a minimum amount of water required for pressing. In wet mixing, first the mix with the raw clay is soaked with water for about 2 days so that fine clay can be distributed uniformly all through the batch composition and then the mix was charged in pan mixer or pug mill and mixed for few hours. The mixed composition is allowed to be aged for days in a cool cellar for better aging and increased uniform plasticity.

The shaping of the mixed refractory compositions is done by hand molding, pneumatic ramming, or pressing. Depending on the shaping process, the moisture content of the mixed composition may vary between 4 and 12 wt%. Lower moisture content results in high molding pressure and higher moisture content leads to a higher chance of slumping. Also low-pressure products are less dense and have lower strength compared to dry pressed products. Again hand molding and ramming processes produce non-uniform pressure during shaping and results in non-uniform properties. The size of these low-pressure products may also not be appropriate due to high shrinkage, and so higher-sized products are made and sintered, which are cut to get proper dimensions. Again pressing method allows a very high production rate but cannot produce any complicatedly shaped and large sized product. The increasing demand for greater productivity results in most of the products shaped by the pressing method, employing various types of presses, including hydraulic presses. A uniform and homogeneous structure, better compaction, higher density, improved strength, etc. are the characteristics of these products. A compaction pressure of 50–80 MPa is used for the fireclay refractories. Excessive pressure may result in cracks in the fired products. Again the fireclay raw particles are very fine and result in high shrinkage both after drying and firing. Hence, the dimensions of the molds and dies are to be adjusted accordingly.

Shaped articles are dried before firing to remove mainly the physically absorbed moisture, and drying is critical for fireclay bodies. Very slow drying is done with no direct heating of the surface in the initial periods. Very fine clay particles may shrink unevenly and may result in non-uniform drying and non-uniform shrinkage that can result in cracks. This is more important for high moisture containing shapes and about 1–4 days of natural drying in open air (not in direct sunlight) is done before a final drying in the ovens or driers. Hot air or waste heat is used in the driers to reach the highest temperature of 150–250°C and a total drying time of 24–200 h is used depending on the moisture content and grog amount.

After drying, the dried shapes are fired in batch (down draft, chamber kiln) or continuous kilns (tunnel kiln). Firing is done slowly to accommodate the structural changes that occur within fireclay, reactions and phase formations, and shrinkage. The total firing schedule is classified into five stages depending on the changes occurring within the refractory being fired and the temperature zone.

In the first stage, from room temperature to about 500°C, most of the moisture is removed from the shapes. Any remaining physically absorbed water is expelled around 150–200°C and the chemically absorbed water is removed around 400–450°C. This stage is called "steaming" or "smoking" and steam or smoke is observed to be coming out from the furnace during this period. Steaming is continued for about 20–24 h. All the moisture, present as physical or chemical water, is removed, and the raw clay undergoes a irreversible structural change. It becomes an anhydrous aluminosilicate, which is termed as metakaolin. Next, the second stage is termed as "decomposition," associated with various decompositions and reactions that occur within the fireclay, mainly due to the presence of the impurities. This stage continues up to about 900°C for about 20–24 h. Decompositions of various carbonates (calcium, magnesium), sulfates (iron, calcium), and sulfides (iron) occur during this temperature range, and any free organic mass is finally removed, and any free carbon or sulfur will be oxidized. The third stage is named as "full firing" where no such decomposition occurs, and not much structural change occurs within the refractory. The only major change that occurs in this stage is the decomposition of metakaolin to form mullite and excess silica. This reaction is an exothermic one and results in the evolution of heat. This stage is considered to about 1300°C and lasts for up to 36 h. Above 1300°C, liquid phase is formed due to the presence of various impurities and their reactions with the silicates. This fourth stage is known as the "incipient fusion." In this stage, initially mullite starts crystallizing, and clay particles get hardened. Then the liquid phase helps in enhancing sintering and fills up the gaps between the hard grog particles. The pores are filled with the liquid phase, shrinkage occurs, and a compact hard, dense mass is produced. This stage may continue up to 1500°C, and this is the last stage of heating. Next the refractories are cooled, and the stage is called "cooling or annealing." Slow cooling is done to crystallize the liquid phase and enhance the strength of the refractory. The highest temperature of firing is above the usual application temperature of the refractories to avoid any further shrinkage (PLCR) during use. Also, a higher rate of heating or cooling may be adapted for the refractories having high grog content. Compositions with lesser amount of grog have more amount of finer raw clay, which results in higher shrinkage.

Lower heating rates are used for refractories containing lesser grog, as they undergo higher shrinkage. After firing, the fireclay refractories consist of mullite, cristobalite, residual quartz, and glass. In fired bricks, the mineral components are not present in an equilibrium condition. Only after the installation and use of the fireclay refractories in the furnace, different phases present in the refractory and their amounts change due to high temperature and approach the equilibrium conditions. At higher temperatures and longer holding periods, the mullite content changes little, whereas the content of cristobalite and quartz declines and disappears totally at 1400–1500°C. The fireclay bricks then consist only of mullite and a viscous glass, which mainly consists of silica, some alumina, and alkalis and other fluxing agents formed out of the impurities present in the composition. Overfired refractories may deform due to the presence of excess liquid phase. Underfired refractories will have lower strength and can be fired again for realizing the properties. Fast firing may result in "black heart," a defect due to insufficient supply of oxygen for combustion and decompositions inside the refractory during firing, causing rejection of the refractory.

7.5 CLASSIFICATIONS AND PROPERTIES

Refractories that are made by using fireclay is termed as fireclay refractory. The fireclay being a natural material and a clay of secondary origin varies widely in composition and properties. These variations are prominent among different sources. The Al_2O_3 content in naturally occurring fireclay varies between 25% and 45% and the rest being silica as the major component with impurities. Hence, the refractory made from fireclay also has varying properties depending on the alumina and impurities content. The usefulness of fireclay refractories is largely due to the presence of mineral mullite (containing 72% Al_2O_3), which forms during firing and is characterized by high refractoriness and low thermal expansion. In general, higher the alumina content in fireclay better will be the high-temperature properties. Hence, fireclay refractories are mainly classified according to the alumina content, and the properties also vary with the classification. The nomenclature is referred to the "heat duty" of the refractory, which indicates the temperature withstanding capability of the material in qualitative terms. Higher alumina content allows the material to withstand higher temperature (increases fusion/liquidus temperature), thus improving all the high-temperature properties. Table 7.1 shows the properties of different fireclay refractories. The nomenclature and the details of the fireclay refractories are as follows.

TABLE 7.1   Properties of Fireclay Refractories as per Their Heat Duty (Al_2O_3 Content)

Properties	Heat Duty			
	Super	High	Moderate	Low
Al_2O_3%, min	40	38	30	25
Fe_2O_3%	1.0–1.5	1.5–2.0	2.0–2.5	2.5–3.0
Size tolerance	1	2	2	2.5
Apparent porosity (%), max	20	25	26	28
Cold crushing strength (MPa), min	20	25	27	22
PCE (ASTM) No, min	33	32	30	23
RUL, Ta°C, Min	1450	1400	1370	1340
PLCR	0.4 at 1450°C	1.5 at 1450°C	1.0 at 1350°C	

7.5.1 Super Heat Duty (Al$_2$O$_3$ Content ~40%–45%)

Super heat duty fireclay refractories have an alumina content of minimum 40 wt% and show good strength and refractoriness, high volume stability at high temperatures, and superior thermal shock resistances. Their refractoriness is close to 1800°C and has an RUL value of 1450°C. Higher alumina content requires a higher temperature of firing for proper densification and the high-temperature firing enhances the high-temperature strength, stabilizes their volume and mineral composition, increases their resistance to corrosive agents, and makes them highly resistant to disintegration by carbon monoxide gas.

7.5.2 High Heat Duty (Al$_2$O$_3$ Content 35%–40%)

These refractories have an alumina content of about 38% (35%–40%) with a refractoriness around 1700°C and RUL value of 1400°C. They are important for their greater resistance to thermal shock and used mainly in those linings operated at moderate temperatures over long periods of time but subject to frequent shutdowns (thermal shocks).

7.5.3 Medium Heat Duty (Al$_2$O$_3$ Content 30%–35%)

Medium duty fireclay refractories contain a minimum of 30 wt% alumina and have refractoriness around 1650°C with RUL about 1370°C. Due to strong bonding from the liquid phase, these refractories can withstand abrasion better.

7.5.4 Low Heat Duty (Al$_2$O$_3$ Content 25%–30%)

Low heat duty fireclay refractories have an alumina content of about 25%–30% with a refractoriness around 1600°C and RUL of 1340°C. They are mainly important as backup bricks to support many high-temperature applications.

7.5.5 Semisilica

Semisilica fireclay refractories contain 18%–25% alumina and 65%–80% silica, with a low content of alkalis and other impurities. They are also considered in some cases as a classification of fireclay refractories. They have a refractoriness of 1650°C and RUL of ~1400°C. These refractories have less shrinkage and PLCR values and also have excellent load-bearing strength and volume stability at relatively high temperatures.

The properties of fireclay refractories depend on the amount and type of clay and grog used, amount of alumina and other impurities present in the composition, and types of processing involved. Impurities like alkalis and alkaline earth oxides, iron oxide, and titania react with the silicate phases and reduce the liquidus temperature of the compositions; thus, they affect the high-temperature properties like refractoriness, RUL, shrinkage, etc. The softening behavior of the fireclay refractory is dependent on the amount and the composition of the glassy phase. The moisture content used for shaping the refractories affect the properties by the creation of pores. The amount of raw clay also affects the shrinkage and amount of moisture required for processing. They, in turn, affect the properties of the fired refractories.

As silica is a major component, fireclay refractories have a slightly acidic character. Hence, fireclay refractories are weak against any basic slag, fume, fluxes, and environments. Compact and less porous microstructure of the refractories is stronger against corrosive attacks. Again with mullite being a major phase in the fired refractory, which has a very low thermal expansion characteristics, fireclay refractories also show relative low thermal expansion properties and, in turn, produces better thermal shock resistance character. Coarse textured and high grog containing compositions are again have better thermal shock resistance properties than those of fine textured and low grog containing ones.

Resistance against carbon monoxide gas is specially very important for fireclay refractories. The details have been discussed in Chapters 3 and 4. Fireclay refractories must have low iron content for the application in the stack area of blast furnaces so that they are strong against such degradation.

7.6 APPLICATION OF FIRECLAY BRICKS

The history of refractories indicates that initiation of these materials started with fireclay-based refractories. With the advancement of human civilization, the use of fireclay-based refractories have increased tremendously and until the early of the nineteenth century, it was the most used refractory material. But with the advancement of science and technology and specific demand for refractory properties for specific application areas, slowly and gradually the use of fireclay refractory has reduced. Also, fireclay refractories are acidic in nature, which also restricts its wide applicability in other environments. But still being a comparatively cheap refractory, it is the most common preferred item for any low-temperature applications.

Other than the application environment, the use of fireclay refractories is influenced by several other parameters, like the temperature of applications, load and strength factor, volume stability, etc. The major application areas of fireclay refractories are as follows.

Upper stack of blast furnace: This application does not demand a very high quality refractory as temperature varies between 300°C and 800°C (as shown in Figure 6.3). Hence the common and economic fireclay refractories are suitable for such application. But the critical part is its carbon monoxide environment. Fireclay refractories are suitable for such applications with a maximum Fe_2O_3 content of 1.5%. Depending on the temperature of application area, the alumina content may vary between 35% and 45%.

Hot blast stove: Refractories used in this application require high creep resistance, volume stability, and thermal shock resistance (as shown in Figure 5.5). Low creep fireclay refractories with alumina content around 40%–45% and iron oxide below 2% are used.

Cement rotary kiln: Fireclay refractories are suitable for preheater cyclones, preheating zones, calcination zone, etc., for cement rotary kilns (as shown in Figure 6.3). Temperature varies in these zones from about 300°C to 1100°C and depending on the temperature, the alumina content varies between 25% and 45%, and iron oxide is restricted below 2.5%.

Glass tank furnace: Fireclay refractories are used in the different application of glass industries. Due to high creep resistance up to about 1300°C and excellent thermal shock resistance, they are the preferred choice for checker work of the regenerators of glass tank furnace (except top part), and 40%–45% alumina-containing fireclay with iron oxide <1.2% is useful for regenerators wall and rider arch applications (as shown in Figure 6.3). Similar alumina content with iron oxide content of ~2% is useful for regenerator wall, lower bottom layer, and backup of melting tank.

Baking furnace of aluminum industries: These furnaces are large in structure, built underground with a floating foundation and are made up of several pits or cells. High grog fireclay refractories with alumina content 40%–45% and iron oxide ~2% are used in the flue duct. Depending on the temperature and service conditions, back up walls and head walls are lined with fireclay refractories with alumina 35%–40% and iron oxide up to 2.5%.

Metal casting: Fireclay refractories are also used in steel and metal casting industries, mainly as a funnel, runner, cast pipe, center brick, end runner brick, and ingot mold bottom plate. Refractories containing 30%–40% Al_2O_3 are used for these applications.

Other than the above applications, fireclay refractories are also used in heat recovery systems of different industries (regenerators and recuperators), annealing, and reheating furnaces of steel industries, carbon roasting furnaces, sugar industries, and all the typical and low temperature applications like fireplaces, ovens, flue lines, chimney linings, etc. (Figure 7.1).

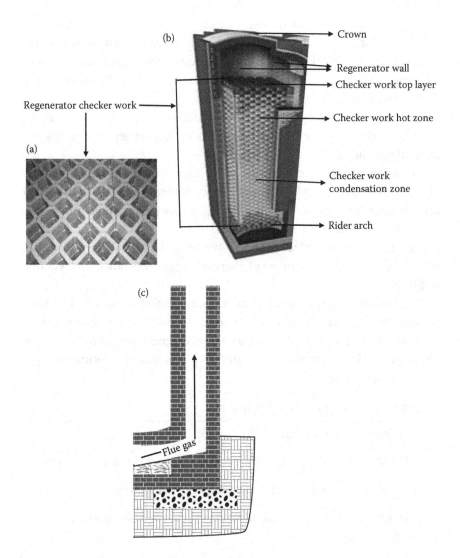

FIGURE 7.1 Applications of fireclay refractories: (a) specific stacking of fireclay refractories in regenerator, (b) regenerator with the stacked checker work, and (c) chimney.

7.7 SUMMARY

Fireclay refractory is the oldest refractory and one of the most widely practiced refractory material.

Natural fireclay is the main raw material for this refractory. Fireclay is a secondary clay commonly found close to coal belts and often with less crystalline water due to partial natural firing from the coal volatile matters.

Very fine particles cause high shrinkage and cracking of the fired refractory. Hence a prefired clay mass, grog, is used as an antishrinkage material to avoid these shortcomings. The addition of grog also provides advantages like enhancement of density, strength, and reduction in water demand during mixing.

The firing of fireclay refractories is little critical due to the presence of various moisture, gas evolution, and structural changes. It also takes a long firing schedule.

Commonly fireclay refractories are of four different types depending upon the heat duty (maximum application temperature) and are classified according to the alumina content. The higher the amount of alumina, better are the high-temperature properties.

Generally, fireclay refractories are medium dense, medium strength, little acidic in nature with good thermal shock resistance and volume stability.

Fireclay refractories are most commonly preferred for any low-temperature application due to its cheapness. The most preferred application areas are blast furnace stack, hot blast stove, regenerator and recuperators, aluminum baking furnaces, preheater cyclones, and preheating zones of cement rotary kilns.

QUESTIONS AND ASSIGNMENTS

1. Discuss the mineral fireclay.

2. What are the advantages and disadvantages of fireclay as refractory?

3. What is grog and what are advantages of using grog?

4. Describe in detail the manufacturing technique for making fireclay refractories.

5. Discuss the firing of fireclay refractories.

6. Detail the classification of fireclay refractories with the property variation.

7. Discuss the properties of fireclay refractories.

8. Briefly mention the applications of fireclay refractories.

9. Describe the variation in properties of fireclay with the alumina content.

BIBLIOGRAPHY

1. J. H. Chesters, *Refractories—Production and Properties*, Woodhead Publishing Ltd., Cambridge, UK, 2006.
2. P. P. Budnikov, *The Technology of Ceramics and Refractories*, 4th edn., translated by E. Arnold, *Scripta Technica*, The MIT Press, Cambridge, MA, 2003.
3. A. R. Chesti, *Refractories: Manufacture, Properties and Applications*, Prentice-Hall of India, New Delhi, 1986.
4. *Refractories Handbook*, The Technical Association of Refractories, Japan, 1998.
5. *Harbison-Walker Handbook of Refractory Practice*, Harbison-Walker, PA, 2005.
6. D. N. Nandi, *Handbook on Refractories*, Tata McGraw-Hill, India, New Delhi, 1987.

CHAPTER 8

Magnesia Refractories

8.1 INTRODUCTION

The major part of the total refractory produced, about 75%, is used in iron and steel industries. Again the steel industries are working in a basicity condition since long and to make the refractories chemically compatible basic refractories are a must for metal contact areas in steel manufacturing plants. Alumina, being neutral in character, survives well in the iron and steel industries, but as it shows little acidic character at high temperatures, and in certain areas it reacts with lime, present in the slag, very fast and deteriorates the refractory lining. Hence, use of basic refractories is of prime importance, especially in those liquid contact areas having high basicity.

From the basicity point of view, lime, CaO (melting point 2570°C), is the best among the oxides, and the lime refractory may be the most suitable for any high temperature and high basicity applications. Also, lime is abundantly available in nature, calcium being the fifth most abundant element in earth's crust. But among all these positive qualities, only the problem of hydration has restricted lime to be commercially successful as refractories. Lime has very high hydration character, and it reacts with the moisture, present in air, instantaneously forming calcium hydroxide [CaO + H$_2$O = Ca(OH)$_2$] even in sintered or a fused form. This hydration causes expansion, cracks the shapes, and makes powdered hydroxide material form sintered shapes. Plenty of research work has been done to restrict or reduce the hydration character of lime but the commercial and economical process to do the same is yet to be established, and lime refractories are not being practiced commercially and widely.

From the basicity and availability point of view, next to lime comes magnesia. Magnesia or magnesium oxide (MgO) is a white, little hygroscopic, solid mineral, which is available in the natural state in limited amount with a mineralogical name "periclase." It also absorbs moisture from the environment and forms magnesium hydroxide [$MgO + H_2O = Mg(OH)_2$], but this reaction is relatively sluggish compared to lime and high sintered and fused products have very limited hydration tendencies.

In the earth's crust, magnesium (Mg) is the eighth most abundant element and constitutes about 2% of the earth's crust. Although magnesium is available in more than 60 minerals, only dolomite, magnesite, brucite, carnallite, and olivine are of commercial importance due to their concentration level. Again, magnesium is the third most available element dissolved in seawater, with a concentration averaging 0.13%. Magnesium and magnesium-bearing compounds can be produced from seawater and brines of wells and lakes.

A relatively high basic character with a wide natural availability coupled with limited hydration character has made magnesia the most suitable material for basic refractories. In most of the application areas in highly basic environments, especially the slag contact areas of steelmaking and steel-processing applications, refractories containing magnesia is most suitable and being practiced globally.

8.2 RAW MATERIALS AND SOURCES

Magnesia refractories are manufactured from various raw material sources, which are described in the following.

8.2.1 Magnesite

Magnesite ($MgCO_3$) is the naturally occurring carbonate of magnesium and the most common source of magnesia used for many important industrial applications. The term "magnesite" literally refers only to the naturally occurring mineral, however in common usage, it is being used for the end products as well (like magnesite refractories which contain MgO). Theoretically, it contains 47.6% MgO and rest of it is carbonates. It is available in two different physical forms in nature, namely (i) macrocrystalline and (ii) cryptocrystalline. Cryptocrystalline magnesite is generally of a higher purity than macrocrystalline ore but tends to occur in smaller deposits than the macrocrystalline form. It is commonly associated with ferrous carbonate and magnesium silicates (like serpentine and olivines).

At high temperatures, $MgCO_3$ decomposes into magnesium oxide and carbon dioxide:

$$MgCO_3 \rightarrow MgO + CO_2$$

The decomposition starts at a temperature of around 350°C, but heating to around 900°C is required to obtain the complete oxide phase due to interfering readsorption of the liberated carbon dioxide. This low-temperature calcined MgO can be hydrated from the atmospheric moisture to form magnesium hydroxide. To reduce or avoid hydration, calcination is done between 1100°C and 1300°C to get caustic magnesia, obtained in a loose form. Caustic calcined MgO is characterized by high chemical reactivity, fine crystal size, high porosity, and low bulk density. Caustic calcined MgO occasionally finds use in the metallurgical industry as slag conditioner but is rarely employed in refractory products and never as a major aggregate ingredient. It is used in agricultural and industrial applications, like feed supplement to cattle, fertilizers, electrical insulations, industrial fillers, and in flue gas desulfurization.

The calcined magnesia that is fired to a very high temperature to make it completely non-reactive is called dead burnt magnesia (DBM). Before dead burning, magnesite was beneficiated by conventional methods (optical sorting, heavy media separation, and magnetic separation) or by processes like floatation to reduce the impurity content. The calcined form of magnesia is briquetted and dead burnt in a rotary kiln or shaft kiln at temperatures around 1900–2000°C. The MgO content in DBM varies between 85% and 98%, and the major impurities are SiO_2, CaO, Fe_2O_3, etc. DBM is characterized by low chemical reactivity, large crystal size, low porosity, and high bulk density. Magnesia is the highest melting common refractory oxide and is the most suitable heat containment material for high-temperature processes in the steel industry. And DBM is the most widely and commonly used sources of magnesia. Although China is the largest producer of DBM, there are significant resources in North Korea, Turkey, Austria, Slovakia, Brazil, Russia, Spain, and Australia.

8.2.2 Fused Magnesia

Fused magnesia is produced in an electric arc furnace using high-grade magnesite or calcined magnesia as raw materials. About 12 h is required for the fusion process at temperatures above the melting point of 2825°C and then it is cooled very slowly. The process promotes the growth of periclase crystals to very large sizes (even greater than 1000 microns compared to 100 microns for dead burned magnesia) with a density approaching the theoretical maximum of 3.58 g/cc. The resulting product is then crushed and ground to get the desired fractions. Fused magnesia is superior to dead burnt magnesia in strength, abrasion resistance, and chemical stability. Fused magnesite is manufactured in the locations where natural magnesite is in abundance, for example, China, Turkey, and Australia.

The addition of fused magnesia grains can significantly enhance the performance and durability of the basic refractories. The primary reasons are higher density, large periclase crystal size, and realignment of accessory silicates. Increased crystal size reduces the grain boundary, reducing the area for any chemical reaction, and thus increases the corrosion resistance. Also, as the magnesia is fused above 2800°C, it becomes immune to react at any lower temperature and has lower porosity levels. So fused products have lesser tendency to react in any environment. Refractory-grade fused magnesia is normally characterized by

- High magnesia content (minimum 97% MgO)

- Low silica content (lime to silica ratio >2)

- Densities ~3.50 g/cc or more

- Large periclase crystal sizes (1000 microns minimum)

Due to its relatively high chemical stability, strength, resistance to abrasion, and excellent corrosion resistance, refractory-grade fused magnesia is used in high wear areas in steelmaking, like the molten metal and slag contact areas. Fused magnesia also has high thermal conductivity due to higher density values. But the main constraints for making fused MgO are the size and number of electric arc furnaces and the cost of energy. The manufacturing of fused magnesia is highly power intensive with electricity consumption varying between 3500 and 4500 kWh/ton.

8.2.3 Seawater Magnesia

Magnesium is present as a soluble salt in seawater which contains about 1.3×10^{-3} kg/L Mg^{2+} ions in combination with chloride and sulfate ions. When it is represented in the form of an oxide (MgO), this amount becomes ~2×10^{-3} kg/L. Theoretically, this can be extracted easily by the addition of a suitable alkaline compounds in seawater. The first large-scale commercial plant for producing refractory-grade magnesia was built at

Hartlepool, by the Steetley Company in 1938 using seawater and dolomite. Because of their consistent composition and quality, seawater magnesia is preferred compared to natural magnesia. The impurities, present as trace elements in seawater, are controlled by careful raw material selection. By controlling the preparation and precipitation conditions, the amounts of chloride, sulfate, and other ions can be controlled. Also, certain trace elements are added to this magnesia for the betterment in sintering and properties.

To precipitate out magnesium from seawater, nearly all the processes use lime-bearing compounds, like calcined and hydrated limestone or dolomite. Calcium ion replaces the magnesium ion, combines with the chloride or sulfate anions and gets dissolved as soluble salt whereas magnesium precipitates out in its hydroxide form. In this process, first limestone or dolomite is calcined in a rotary kiln at 1300–1400°C.

$$CaCO_3 = CaO + CO_2$$

$$(Mg, Ca)CO_3 = MgO \cdot CaO + CO_2$$

Then the calcined product, lime or doloma is hydrated:

$$CaO + H_2O = Ca(OH)_2$$

$$(Mg, Ca)O + H_2O = (Mg, Ca)(OH)_2$$

This hydrated material is then reacted with seawater stored in big tanks with agitation, which results in the following chemical reactions:

$$MgCl_2(\text{from seawater}) + Ca(OH)_2 = Mg(OH)_2$$
$$+ CaCl_2(\text{dissolves in seawater})$$

$$MgCl_2(\text{from seawater}) + (Ca, Mg)(OH)_2 = 2Mg(OH)_2$$
$$+ CaCl_2(\text{dissolves in seawater})$$

$$MgSO_4(\text{from seawater}) + Ca(OH)_2 = Mg(OH)_2$$
$$+ CaSO_4(\text{dissolves in seawater})$$

$$MgSO_4(\text{from seawater}) + (Ca, Mg)(OH)_2 = 2Mg(OH)_2$$
$$+ CaSO_4(\text{dissolves in seawater})$$

$Mg(OH)_2$ precipitates out from the water and settles down at the bottom of the tanks with the spent seawater flowing over the top. A flocculent is used to make the settling process more efficient. Part of the slurry is sent back to the reactor to act as a seeding material, and the rest goes to secondary thickeners, where the precipitate is further thickened before filtration. Finally, the slurry is filtered on rotary vacuum disk filters and additions (may be lime, silica, and iron) are made to control the ratios of the impurities and properties enhancement of magnesia. The filter cake, containing about 50% solids, is then either fed directly into the rotary kiln and fired above 1900°C or calcined first around 1100°C then cooled, pelletized, and sintered in the shaft or rotary kilns above 1800°C.

Very high temperature (over 1800°C) is used for sintering (dead burning) of magnesium oxide results in the formation of larger periclase (MgO) crystals. The kilns transform low-density magnesium oxide into high-density sinters, which has a density of about 3.4 g/cm^3. This product has a buff-brown color and is chemically unreactive. The sintered magnesia produced through this process can also have varying MgO contents, between ~90% and 98%; however, if high-purity magnesia source is used in this process, then the products can have MgO contents in excess of 99%. Also for making high-purity magnesia, calcined dolomite is not used as natural dolomite contains about 1.3% Fe_2O_3, which will impart higher iron impurities in the product.

The main impurities of seawater magnesia are lime, silica, boron oxide, etc. Calcium bicarbonate present in seawater precipitates out as calcium carbonate on reaction with calcium hydroxide

$$[Ca(HCO_3)_2 + Ca(OH)_2 = 2CaCO_3 + 2H_2O],$$

which remains as CaO impurity in the sintered product. Acid pretreatment of seawater can reduce this lime impurity. Also, any unconverted hydrated calcined lime or dolomite used may result in lime impurity. Most of the silica impurity comes from the sand suspended in seawater. Boron is present in small amounts in seawater as boric acid (seawater contains 15 ppm, expressed as B_2O_3). The precipitates of magnesium hydroxides have a high capacity for absorbing boron and the final concentration in the oxide can be as high as 0.4%. This boron contamination can be reduced by using an excess of lime but may result in excess lime content in the product. Also, removal of boron can be done during the dead-burning stage by volatilization. This volatilization rate can be accelerated by the addition of certain alkali metal salts, for example, potassium hydroxide. The presence of boron in magnesia is highly detrimental for its high-temperature properties as it produces very low melting magnesium borate phases.

Due to the presence of different mineral salts, the specific gravity of seawater is higher and varies between 1.02 and 1.03. The highest concentration of mineral salts is available in the water of dead-sea, where the water has a specific gravity of 1.24. Due to the high concentration of minerals, many of the seawater magnesia manufacturing plants are located near the dead-sea and countries like Israel and Jordan are its major producers. Again as the river water has a much lower salt concentration, the river-connected sea areas are not a good option for making seawater magnesia.

8.2.4 Magnesia from Natural Brine Source

Magnesia is also produced from brine solution available in the surface (lakes), subsurface, and subterrain deposits. The composition and concentration of the brine depend on the chemistry and soluble mineral percentage of the surrounding salt-bearing rocks. Naturally occurring subsurface brines are available in porous sandstones and other porous rocks that support the composition. Generally, the concentration of magnesium ion in brine is much higher than seawater, and so the amount of water required to be treated is much lesser than seawater plants. Hence, the same capacity magnesia-producing plant requires much smaller tanks and other processing equipment. Most important sources of subsurface brine are the Nederland and the United States (Mississippian and Pennsylvanian beds, Michigan, etc.).

Lake and well sources of brine are easy ones as the extraction is not so complicated, and involves only the pumping of the solution to the processing plant. However, the underground recovery is a complicated process. Leaching or solution mining of the salt available under the earth using drilling or recovery technology is used as practiced in oil and gas industries. A wide vertical bore well is first drilled from the surface to the deposit. Several concentric tubes or casing are used for the liquid flow to and from the different layers of the deposit source. Water is pumped in which dissolves the salt present underneath, and the solution comes out to the top under the pressure of incoming water.

The brine solution thus obtained is processed in the similar way as that of the seawater, and the rest process is exactly similar to that of the seawater magnesia. However, composition and purity of the final magnesia vary from seawater products due to many impurity salts dissolved in a brine solution, coming from the surrounding rocks of the brine source.

8.2.5 Characteristic of the Raw Materials Affecting the Refractory

The important characteristics of the magnesia raw materials that affect the properties of the final refractory are purity, impurity types and content, crystallite size, density, etc. It is the overall purity of the raw material that plays an important role in determining the MgO content of the final refractory and judges the suitability for a specific application. The MgO content of an aggregate, by and large, determines the slag resistance of the refractory. Again impurities, depending on the type and amount, form low melting liquid phases during use at high temperatures. These liquids when present in-between the grains slide them and finally results in degradation of the high-temperature strength. Also, the liquids help corrosive slags to invade the refractory and drastically reduce the corrosion resistance. Impurities that form a liquid phase at lower temperatures are more detrimental and among them SiO_2 and B_2O_3 are important. Among different impurities, SiO_2, CaO, Al_2O_3, Fe_2O_3, and B_2O_3 (in seawater MgO) are important and common. The impurities do not exist separately and affect MgO individually but they are present in combination, and their effect is more detrimental to MgO.

The crystallite size of MgO is an important parameter for the corrosion of the refractory as it determines the available surface area for any reaction. Any corrosion reaction is a surface activity and reduction in the available surface by increasing the crystallite size of magnesia grain will enhance the corrosion resistance. Fused and high fired magnesia are better in corrosion resistance mainly due to their increased crystallite size. Again, the higher density of the starting materials indicates a lower total porosity value (open and closed pores) and reduces the chance of corrosive liquid penetration and corrosion. It is considered that the densest body offers the best resistance to corrosion against slags and is also strongest to resist abrasion. Hence high dense raw materials will result in better properties.

8.3 BRIEF MANUFACTURING TECHNIQUE

Dead burnt or sintered magnesia is used for the manufacturing of the refractories. Fired lumps are crushed and ground to obtain desired size (maximum ~5 mm), and different fractions are used for obtaining the highest compaction density using coarse, medium, and fine fractions. Crushing and grinding may impart impurities like dust and iron particles, which are required to be cleaned before using the fractions in the mixer.

Different fractions are mixed with a bonding material, required to provide bonding between the hard-fired magnesia particles. This bonding material may be clay, sodium silicate, milk of lime, etc. depending on the type of raw materials; impurities present, and the desired properties in the fired refractories. Also, very little (~0.5%) mill scale (a mixture of different iron oxides) is used to enhance the sintering and strength. In certain applications, 5%–6% alumina is also added as a fine material to form magnesium aluminate spinel within the magnesia refractory matrix, especially to improve the thermal shock resistance. The mixture is mixed with 4%–7% of water (sulfite lye is also added for green strength) to obtain proper consistency, uniformity, and suitable plasticity for the subsequent shaping process. Shaping is done in a hydraulic press at a specific pressure of 80–120 MPa. Next the shapes are dried and fired. Drying of magnesia refractories is critical as cracks may occur. Cracks occur due to

1. Use of soft fired magnesia which may hydrate

2. Presence of excessive fines causing shrinkage and hydration

3. High temperature of the drier. Defect and crack-free samples are processed for firing

Firing is done in batch type (chamber) or continuous type (tunnel) kilns. Firing temperature ranges from 1550°C to 1800°C depending upon the purity and impurities present. The higher the temperature better may be the properties as the shrinkage during application will be reduced. A soaking time of about 4–8 h is given at the peak temperature for uniformity in temperature and uniform property development. As per molecular bonding point of view, magnesia has a strong bonding (ionic) character, compared to silica and alumina, so it has a lower diffusivity and poor sinterability. Hence, magnesia sinters poorly and sintering aid (mill scale) is necessary. Iron oxide of mill scale reacts with magnesia and forms magnesioferrite, which is present in between the magnesia grains and helps in bonding between the magnesia grains and improves sintering, densification and strength.

8.4 EFFECT OF LIME:SILICA RATIO

Both lime (CaO) and silica (SiO_2) are common and abundant impurities for magnesia refractories. The presence of lime is not as harmful as most of the impurities because alone it does not degrade the properties of magnesia (as detailed in the phase diagram, described later). But silica, if present, produces low melting silicates and affects the high-temperature properties drastically. Impurities are more effective in finer form, due to the greater reaction from higher surface area and produces liquid phase at low temperatures. So the deterioration in properties starts mainly in the matrix phase. But the deteriorating effect of silica can be controlled by the presence of lime as the reaction products form in the presence of lime are different. Hence the amount of lime present and the ratio of lime-to-silica is important for the properties and performance of the magnesia refractories. Other impurities, commonly iron oxide, also take part in the reactions and form complex compounds.

Again the presence of huge amount of lime can deteriorate the properties due to the hydration tendency of lime. So the presence of lime in magnesia refractories is important and amount of the same is to be controlled depending upon the amount of silica present as an impurity. Table 8.1 details the different ratios of lime:silica and the possible compound formation in the matrix phase and their melting or fusion points. Also Figure 8.1 shows the $CaO-SiO_2$

TABLE 8.1   Effect of Lime Silica Ratio on Compound Formation in Magnesia Refractories

Lime:Silica ($CaO:SiO_2$) Ratio, X				Melting/Fusion Point (°C)
Molar Ratio	Weight Ratio	Possible Phases	Chemical Formula	
$X < 1$	$X < 0.94$	Forsterite	$2MgO \cdot SiO_2$	1890
		Monticelite	$CaO \cdot MgO \cdot SiO_2$	1503
		Magnesio-ferrite	$MgO \cdot Fe_2O_3$	1760
$X = 1$	$X = 0.94$	Monticelite	$CaO \cdot MgO \cdot SiO_2$	1503
		Magnesio-ferrite	$MgO \cdot Fe_2O_3$	1760
$1 < X < 1.5$	$0.94 < X < 1.4$	Merwinite	$3CaO \cdot MgO \cdot 2SiO_2$	1550
		Monticelite	$CaO \cdot MgO \cdot SiO_2$	1503
		Magnesio-ferrite	$MgO \cdot Fe_2O_3$	1760
$X = 1.5$	$X = 1.4$	Merwinite	$3CaO \cdot MgO \cdot 2SiO_2$	1550
		Magnesio-ferrite	$MgO \cdot Fe_2O_3$	1760
$1.5 < X < 2$	$1.4 < X < 1.87$	Merwinite	$3CaO \cdot MgO \cdot 2SiO_2$	1550
		Belite	$2CaO \cdot SiO_2$	2130
		Magnesio-ferrite	$MgO \cdot Fe_2O_3$	1760
$X = 2$	$X = 1.87$	Belite	$2CaO \cdot SiO_2$	2130
		Magnesio-ferrite	$MgO \cdot Fe_2O_3$	1760
$X > 2$	$X > 1.87$	Belite	$2CaO \cdot SiO_2$	2130
		Alite	$3CaO \cdot SiO_2$	2070
		Magnesio-ferrite	$MgO \cdot Fe_2O_3$	1760

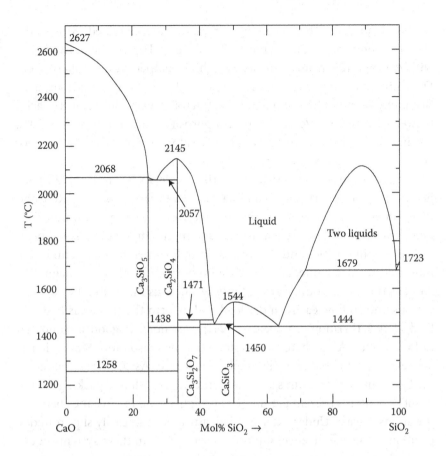

FIGURE 8.1   Phase diagram of lime (CaO)–silica (SiO₂) system.

phase diagram, detailing the compounds present in the system and the liquid phase formation.

It can be seen from the Table 8.1 that the low-melting compounds, namely monticellite and merwinite, form when the ratio is below 2. Also, these two compounds, if present together, can produce liquid phase even at further lower temperature of ~1450°C. Hence, a lime:silica ratio of over 2 is necessary for avoiding any formation of these low-melting compounds.

8.5 CLASSIFICATIONS AND PROPERTIES

Magnesia refractories have periclase as the main constituent with a few compounds based on the impurities present, namely, belite (2CaO SiO₂), alite (3CaO SiO₂), forsterite (2MgO SiO₂), monticellite (CaO · MgO · SiO₂), and some magnesia ferrite. Depending upon the purity and impurities type and quantity, the magnesia refractories are classified. Mostly the classification is based on the purity (% of MgO). Higher the purity better will be properties from corrosion and high-temperature points of view. Depending on the purity, impurity types and processing conditions, density, and porosity values of magnesia refractories vary. Bulk density varies between 2.8 and 3.1 g/cc and apparent porosity in the range of 14%–20%. As sintering is difficult for magnesia, generally the strength values are not very high and vary between 400 and 800 kg/cm^2.

Though magnesia is a very high melting oxide, its strength at high-temperature is not remarkable. Magnesia has a wide gap between its RUL and PCE values in comparison to other refractories, say silica or alumina. The main reason for its low strength values at high temperatures is the presence of the impurities and the formation of low-melting compounds like monticellite, merwinite, and magnesium borate (for seawater magnesia). Also, as these compounds are not highly siliceous in nature, they are low viscous and so flow easily under load and deform the shape easily under load. Hence, thermomechanical properties are not very good as compared to PCE values. Also, there is a crystallographic reason too. Magnesia has a face-centered cubic crystallographic structure. As per crystallography, the face centered structures are having the densest atomic packing. So the number of atoms present per unit cell is highest and the distance between the atoms is least. Under external load, any atom can easily slip from one position to another. Hence, slip occurs very easily in these systems under stressed conditions as the gap between the two slip planes is minimum. Generally, the RUL value of magnesia refractory varies between 1550°C and 1650°C depending on its purity.

Magnesia, being a strong basic material, has a very good corrosion resistance against basic slags and environments. But it is highly vulnerable in any acidic environment. It also shows a very strong resistance against high FeO-containing slags as magnesia can absorb FeO in its structure by forming a solid solution. Slag resistance of magnesia refractories increases with the increase in purity. However, increase in porosity and presence of rough surface cause an increase in slag corrosion.

Magnesia has a high thermal expansion properties and has a coefficient of ~13×10^{-6} °C^{-1}, which is very high among the oxides. Due to expansion properties, magnesia refractories have poor thermal spalling resistance and disintegrate under thermal cycling. Even it is hard to attain 20 thermal cycles (of 1000°C heating and air cooling) for a pure magnesia refractory. It has been observed that (a) prolonged heating at highest temperature to form the maximum extent of periclase and to complete any reaction within the impurities, (b) reduction in FeO content in the composition, and (c) use of fine grinding and high-pressing pressure, resulting in greater sintering, improve the thermal spalling character. Also to improve the thermal spalling character, alumina or chromia is added to form respective spinels, which improves the property.

8.6 EFFECT OF IMPURITIES ON PHASE DIAGRAMS

It has been discussed that magnesia is associated with certain impurities. Natural magnesite source is mainly associated with impurities like CaO, Fe_2O_3 and SiO_2 and seawater source is associated with CaO and harmful B_2O_3. Also to improve the sintering of strongly ionic bonded magnesia, mill scale (mainly Fe_2O_3) is added. Hence, the most common impurities present in magnesia refractories are CaO and Fe_2O_3. Figure 8.2 shows the binary phase diagram of MgO with CaO and Fe_2O_3. It can be seen that the MgO–CaO diagram has no liquid phase below 2370°C, the hence the presence of only CaO does not pose a serious danger for magnesia refractories. Also, a good amount of CaO also goes into the MgO structure forming a solid solution. So from the refractory point of view, CaO alone is not a harmful impurity in magnesia refractories.

Again, the presence of Fe_2O_3 in magnesia forms magnesio-wustite [(Mg, Fe)O] solid solution, in which iron is accommodated in the magnesia structure. Absorption of iron is maximum at around 1720°C and decreases sharply at lower temperatures. Below 1000°C, the presence of iron results in two different compounds: magnesiowustite and magnesio-ferrite ($MgFe_2O_4$). The presence of liquid phase is observed at low temperatures in the very high iron-containing portions, and the melting point of Fe_2O_3 is the minimum temperature for the existence of liquid phase. For magnesia-rich region (which is the case for magnesia refractories), the liquid forms on melting of the magnesiowustite phase, which decreases with an increasing amount of Fe_2O_3. However, the minimum temperature of about 1720°C is reached for a Fe_2O_3 content of more than 65 wt%, which is far higher than any magnesia refractory composition. Hence for a lower amount of Fe_2O_3, the liquid phase formation occurs at very high temperatures and only iron oxide does not affect the properties strongly.

The effect of other harmful impurities is shown in Figure 8.3. It can be seen that in the presence of SiO_2, the liquidus drops sharply and the eutectic forms at about 1840°C. But silica does not make any solid solution with MgO and so even a minute amount of silica will result in the formation of

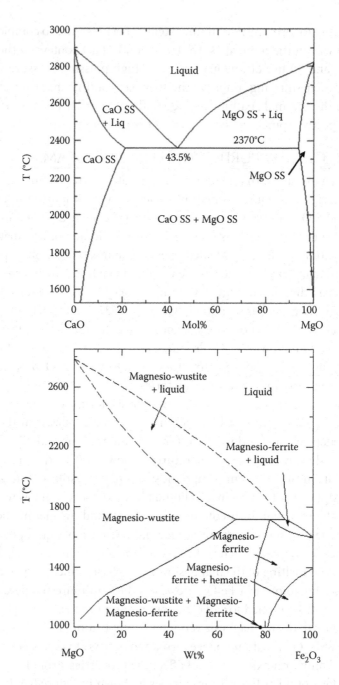

FIGURE 8.2   Phase diagram of magnesia with lime (CaO) and iron oxide (Fe_2O_3).

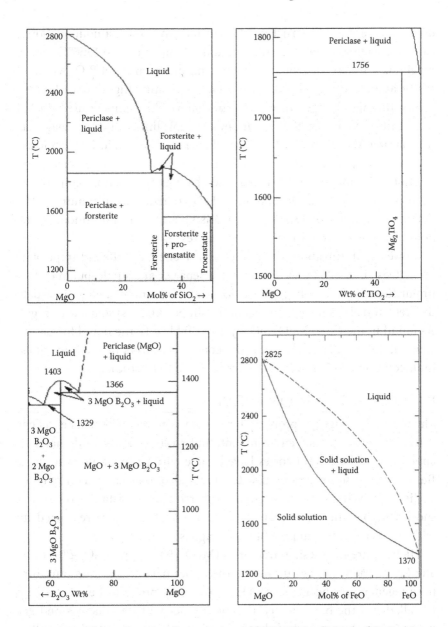

FIGURE 8.3   Phase diagram of magnesia with SiO_2, TiO_2, B_2O_3, and FeO.

a little amount of liquid phase at and above 1840°C. The similar character is also observed in the presence of TiO_2. There is no formation of solid solution between MgO and TiO_2, and any small presence of TiO_2 leads to liquid phase formation with MgO at and above 1756°C. The strongest effect in reducing the liquidus temperature was observed for B_2O_3. Boron also does not enter into the structure of MgO and any minute amount of boron can reduce (at least starts forming) liquidus temperature to 1366°C. Hence magnesia refractories containing even a minute amount of B_2O_3 will have a little amount of liquid phase even at a temperature higher than 1366°C. Hence the high-temperature properties above this temperature will fall drastically. That is why the maximum allowable limit of B_2O_3 in magnesia (in seawater MgO) is 0.01 wt%. Again if iron is present in its bivalent form, that is as FeO, or if FeO comes from slag, then it forms a complete solid solution, with magnesia. In such a case, the liquid formation temperature decreases with increasing amount of FeO content and minimum at the FeO melting point of 1370°C. As FeO is present in minor amounts, the liquid formation occurs at high temperatures.

However, all the above discussion on the effect of different impurities on MgO is done when they are present as separate and single, but in reality, impurities are present in combination and the combined effect is widely different and also severe than that of the simple binary systems with MgO. As found in the $CaO–MgO–SiO_2$ system (Table 8.1), the liquid formation starts at 1503°C. To understand the combined effects of the impurities, multicomponent phase diagrams are required to be studied.

8.7 MAIN APPLICATION AREAS

The most advantageous property for magnesia refractories is its excellent resistance against basic environment, and so it is highly in demand in applications where refractories have basic environments and basic slags. But, there are some serious disadvantages also associated with magnesia like relatively lower hot strength properties, low resistance to thermal shocks, higher thermal expansion, and conductivity have restricted its wide use as a single-component pure magnesia refractory.

Highly pure magnesia refractories (MgO ~95%–97%, CaO ~2%–1.5%, and SiO_2 ~1%–0.5%) are useful for the upper part of the glass tank furnace regenerator checker work. This portion is prone to be attacked by the alkalis of the batch materials, coming out with the flue gas and get deposited on the top part of checker work. Resistance to alkali and sulfur attack is of prime importance in that region. Also, these type of magnesia refractories are important for the chemical industries where a high basic environment prevails. Incorporation of zirconia (10%–12%) is also done in the glass regenerator applications to improve the abrasion resistance as solid batch materials are discharged at a high speed with the flue gas and abrade the refractory surfaces.

The next-level purity class magnesia refractories (MgO ~95%, CaO ~2%, and SiO_2 ~2%) are used in a lime kiln, where lime stone is calcined, and high basic environments prevail. Magnesia refractory with 92% MgO and impurities about 2% CaO and ~4% SiO_2 are used for the hot metal mixer in the iron and steel industries. Backup of the lining of converters, ladles, and electric arc furnaces of steel industries are done by using relatively less pure magnesia refractories (MgO ~87%, CaO ~2%, and SiO_2 ~6%). Relatively inferior magnesia refractories containing about 50% MgO are used for the reheating furnace hearth applications.

8.8 SUMMARY

Magnesia is the most important basic oxide mainly used as basic refractory. Though lime has higher basicity, but due to hydration tendency, it is not widely practiced commercially.

There are three major raw material sources of magnesia, namely natural magnesia, seawater magnesia, and brine magnesia. Natural magnesite is mainly associated with impurities like lime, silica, and iron oxide. For seawater magnesia, the most harmful impurity is B_2O_3. For brine magnesia, the major impurities are also iron oxide and silica. There is also fused magnesia available, produced by electrofusion route and used to improve the corrosion resistances.

Conventional-shaped refractory manufacturing technique is used for making magnesia refractories, but as magnesia is a strong ionic bonded oxide, its sintering requires higher temperature and mill scale (mainly Fe_2O_3) is added as a sintering aid during mixing.

Among impurities, silica is very common in natural magnesite, which can form low melting impurity phase (silicates) that can strongly deteriorate the high-temperature properties. Hence, it is a practice to have high lime content in magnesia refractory having silica as an impurity. The presence of lime will react with silica, forming high-temperature melting di- and tri-calcium silicates, thus improving the high-temperature properties. So lime to silica ratio is important and is maintained above 2.

Magnesia has relatively higher thermal expansion property, resulting in poor thermal shock resistance. It has very high corrosion resistance against basic slags or environments, but for slags with high FeO, it may form a solid solution and get dissolved in the slag, causing high wear out of the refractory.

It is mostly used in the backup lining of steel converters, steel ladles, electric arc furnaces, top part in the checker work of glass tank furnace regenerators, in lime kilns, etc.

QUESTIONS AND ASSIGNMENTS

1. Why is lime not commonly used in a basic refractory?

2. What are the different raw material sources for magnesia refractories? Discuss them.

3. What are the main impurities present in different raw material sources for magnesia? How do they affect the quality of magnesia?

4. How does lime:silica ratio affect the properties of magnesia refractories?

5. Discuss the manufacturing technique for making magnesia refractories.

6. Discuss why magnesia has much lower thermomechanical properties compared to its PCE.

7. Why is CaO not a harmful impurity for magnesia but SiO_2 and B_2O_3 are?

8. Discuss the main application areas of magnesia refractories.

9. Describe with phase diagram how a magnesia refractory will behave with a slag containing high FeO.

BIBLIOGRAPHY

1. J. H. Chesters, *Refractories—Production and Properties*, Woodhead Publishing Ltd., Cambridge, UK, 2006.
2. P. P. Budnikov, *The Technology of Ceramics and Refractories*, 4th edn., translated by E. Arnold, *Scripta Technica*, The MIT Press, 2003.
3. A. R. Chesti, *Refractories: Manufacture, Properties and Applications*, Prentice-Hall of India, New Delhi, 1986.
4. *Refractories Handbook*, The Technical Association of Refractories, Japan, 1998.
5. *Harbison-Walker Handbook of Refractory Practice*, Harbison-Walker, PA, 2005.
6. Y. Yin and B. B. Argent, The phase diagrams and thermodynamics of the ZrO_2–CaO–MgO and MgO–CaO systems. *Journal of Phase Equilibria*, 14(5), 588–600, 1993.

7. E. Woermann, B. Brezny, and A. Muan, Phase equilibria in the system MgO–iron oxide–TiO$_2$ in air. *American Journal of Science*, 267A, 463–479, 1969.

8. S. Miyagawa, S. Hirano, and S. Somiya, Phase relations in the system MgO-B$_2$O$_3$ and effects of boric oxide on grain growth of magnesia. *Yogyo Kyokaishi*, 80(2), 53–63, 1972.

9. P. Wu, G. Eriksson, A. D. Pelton, and M. Blander, Prediction of the thermodynamic properties and phase diagrams of silicate systems—Evaluation of the FeO–MgO–SiO$_2$ system. *ISIJ International*, 33(1), 26–35, 1993.

10. V. Swamy, S. K. Saxena, and B. Sundman, CALPHAD: Comput. *Coupling Phase Diagrams Thermochemistry*, 18(2), 157–164, 1994.

11. B. Phillips, S. Somiya, and A. Muan, Melting relations of magnesium oxide-iron oxide mixtures in air. *Journal of American Ceramic Society*, 44(4), 167–169, 1961.

12. J. D. Panda, Planned utilization of raw materials for basic refractories. *Proceedings of Indian National Science Academy*, 50A(5), 428–38, 1984.

13. A. S. Bhatti, D. Dollimore, and A. Dyer, Magnesia from seawater: A review. *Clay Minerals*, 19, 865–875, 1984.

14. H. M. Richardson, M. Lester, F. T. Palin, and P. T. A. Hodson, The effect of boric oxide on some properties of magnesia. *Transactions of British Ceramic Society*, 68, 29–31, 1969.

CHAPTER 9

Dolomite Refractories

9.1 INTRODUCTION

From the basicity point of view, lime has an edge over magnesia, but hydration has restricted its success. However, a mixture of lime and magnesia can be used having both the positive and negatives of both the oxides. Hydration tendency of lime is thus reduced with increase basicity for magnesia. Such a natural raw material source is dolomite.

Dolomite is a double carbonate of calcium and magnesium or calcium magnesium carbonate $[CaMg(CO_3)_2]$, occurring naturally in many countries and widely used in many industrial applications. The mineral was first identified by Count Dolomien in 1791 and named after its discoverer. Being a natural mineral usually dolomite contains impurities, chiefly silica, alumina and iron oxide. For commercial purposes, the percentage of combined impurities should not go beyond 7%, above which, it becomes unsuitable for industrial use. High impurity containing dolomite is used only for road ballasts, building stones, flooring chips, etc. For refractory industries, the purer variety of dolomite is used with a min MgO content of 20% and combined CaO + MgO min 52%. Dolomite with lower purity are important for other industries, like iron and steel, ferro-manganese, glass, fertilizer, etc. Table 9.1 gives an idea about the quality of the raw dolomite and their recommended use.

In iron and steel industry dolomite is important as a flux material. Dolomite used in blast furnace, sinter and pellet plants are of relatively inferior quality (MgO min 19% and combined CaO + MgO min 46%) as compared to that used in steel melting shop (MgO min 20% and combined CaO + MgO min 50%). Dolomite is important in iron making and steel

TABLE 9.1 Quality of Raw Dolomite and Recommended Industry for Application

Recommended for	Refractory Industry	Steel Making	Iron Making
(CaO + MgO) Content, % mass, min	52	50	46
CaO content, % mass, min	–	30	–
MgO content, % mass, min	20	20	19
SiO2 content, % mass, max	2	2	–
Total acid insoluble, % mass, max	2	3	8
Alkali content, % mass, max	0.2	0.2	0.2

making processes to produce a highly basic low melting liquid phase that can extract out the gangue (impurity) materials present (silica, alumina, etc.) in iron ore and form the slag easily. For ferro-manganese industry also the dolomite used is of similar quality to steel grade ones (MgO 19%–20%, CaO 28%–30%, SiO_2 2%–5%, and Al_2O_3 2%–2.5%). But for ferro-manganese industries, dolomite should be hard and fine grained because crystalline dolomite gives fritting effect in the furnace. In the glass industry, dolomite is a source of lime, essentially required for the chemical property of glass (corrosion resistant) and MgO source which helps in preventing crystallization. Also dolomite provides low temperature eutectics (due to presence of two basic oxides) with acidic systems (silica in glass) and helps in glass formation. But it must be nearly free from iron or any other coloring oxides. Dolomite used in fertilizer industries is mainly used for soil amendments and must have $MgCO_3$ + $CaCO_3$ min 90% and finer than 2 mm size.

9.2 RAW MATERIALS AND SOURCES

Dolomite is a naturally occurring sedimentary and metamorphic mineral, found as the principal mineral in widely and abundantly available dolostones and meta-dolostones. It is also an important mineral in certain limestones and marbles, where calcite is the principal mineral present. Dolomite is also found as a hydrothermal vein mineral, forming crystals in cavities; and in serpentinites and similar rocks. Theoretically dolomite contains 54.35% $CaCO_3$ and 45.65% $MgCO_3$ and as per oxide contents it has 30.4% CaO, 21.7% MgO and 47.9% CO_2. In nature, considerable variations in the composition of dolomite relating to lime and magnesia percentages are found. When the percentage of $CaCO_3$ increases by 10% or moreover the theoretical composition, the mineral is termed "calcitic dolomite," "high-calcium dolomite," or "lime-dolomite." With the decrease in percentage of $MgCO_3$, it is called "dolomitic limestone." When the $MgCO_3$ content is between 5% and 10%, it is called "magnesian limestone," and when it is up to 5%, then it is considered as limestone for all purposes in trade and commercial parlance. Dolomite usually contains impurities, chiefly silica, alumina, and iron oxide.

At the present time, dolomite does not form on the surface of the earth; yet massive layers of dolomite as dolostones are very common in ancient rocks. Dolomite is rarely found in modern sedimentary environments but the rock record. They can be geographically extensive and even up to few hundred meters thick. Most of the rocks that are rich in dolomite were originally deposited as calcium carbonate muds and post-depositionally altered by magnesium-rich pore water to form dolomite. Over the time, built-up pressure transformed the mixed composition into dolomite. Eventually, the pressure becomes so great that the mixture hardens into a rock with a high amount of foliation. There is also a high magnesium content to the rock, which is due to magnesium replacement for limestone.

Although rocks containing dolomite are found all over the world, the most important availability of dolomite are located in the Midwestern United States; Ontario, Canada; Switzerland; Pamplona, Spain; Mexico, etc.

9.3 MANUFACTURING PROCESS

Dolomite is a double carbonate which on heating decomposes completely above 900°C. The product resulting from this relatively low-temperature calcination is highly porous and reactive and is known as "calcinated dolomite." This is also termed as "doloma."

$$CaMg(CO_3)_2 = CaO \cdot MgO + 2CO_2$$

This calcined dolomite (or doloma) is also fired for dead burning at high temperatures and contains theoretically 58% of CaO and about 42% of MgO. The presence of free CaO absorbs moisture from the environment and causes hydration.

$$CaO + H_2O = Ca(OH)_2$$

This reaction is associated with volumetric expansion which causes the materials to break down to powder form (hydration/slaking). Hence, any refractory manufactured from the material will also undergo the same hydration process and will shatter. Thus, the doloma is unstable even after dead burning. This hydration may be restricted by converting the lime part of dolomite into an hydraulically inactive silicate phase or some other compounds having a high softening point too. Silica is added to convert the CaO into calcium silicates. Mono-calcium silicate is avoided for its low softening point (~1540°C), but di- and tri-calcium silicates are allowed to form in the composition (due to their high temperature softening character) by reacting all the CaO in the dolomite composition with silica (present in dolomite and added separately). Conversion of CaO to high temperature calcium silicates (mainly di-calcium silicate, preferred due to its high melting point) prevents any hydration, and the final doloma is non-hydratable and stable. This type of calcined product is termed as "stabilized dolomite" and the process is called stabilization. But di-calcium silicates have different crystallographic/polymorphic forms that change during heating and cooling and due to the great difference in the specific gravity of these polymorphic phases, there are huge volumetric changes that cause shattering of the shapes. Phase inversion of di-calcium silicate from its beta to gamma phase during cooling at ~675°C results in a volume expansion of ~10%. This expansion is sudden during cooling and causes cracking and shattering of the refractory. To avoid such disintegration Fe_2O_3 is added that restricts the formation of gamma phase and stabilize the beta phase of di-calcium silicate. This conversion is highly vulnerable from the volumetric expansion point of view, and Fe_2O_3 prevents the same. The addition of boron and phosphate based compounds also help in stabilization of dolomite. But due to the presence high amount of impurity phases like silica, iron oxide, etc. low melting compounds form in doloma due to the reaction between these additions and CaO and MgO of doloma. Hence, the stabilization of dolomite is good for hydration resistance but parallelly results in poor high-temperature properties.

To reduce this deterioration in high-temperature properties, the concept of stabilization is modified to partial stabilization in which much lower amount of silica is added to react with CaO of doloma just to convert the surface of the doloma to di/tri-calcium silicates. As hydration is a surface activity at low temperatures, the coating of silicates on the surface protects the material from hydration and also the properties are not strongly affected. Instead of addition of silica, serpentine ($3MgO\ 2SiO_2\ 2H_2O$) is also used to form high temperature silicates with excess MgO in the composition.

$$6(CaO \cdot MgO) + 3(MgO\ 2SiO_2\ 2H_2O) = 2(3CaO \cdot SiO_2) + 9MgO + 2H_2O$$

Calcining and dead burning of dolomite (containing stabilizers like silica) are done in a rotary kiln or shaft kiln. The dolomite stone is crushed to desired sizes as per the kiln type and size and then washed to make it free from impurity particles, like clay. The total treatment process to get the sintered doloma grains may be divided into four steps. They are drying (to remove external and any internal moisture), calcination (to remove the gaseous material like CO_2), firing or dead burning (to get dense sintered aggregates with reduced porosity, temperature depends on the composition and desired product) and cooling.

As the process of stabilization basically imparts impurity and a compromise is required between hydration tendency and high temperature properties, new techniques have come up to produce very high fired doloma aggregates to reduce hydration tendency and processing them fast to convert to refractory bricks and cover them to avoid any hydration. In one technique, termed as single pass process, where the dolomite is passed through the kiln once only, involves very high temperature dead burning of the natural purer dolomite, above 1800°C, to make the aggregate immune and increase the grain size to reduce the hydration tendency. Also processing the aggregates to make bricks in a fast process (brick manufacturer itself makes the aggregate in the same site to avoid any time delay for transportation). In another route, termed as double pass process, a two stage firing is involved with a pelletization process in between. In the first firing, dolomite is calcined to produce active oxide which is pelletized and fired at high temperatures to immune the material. These firing temperatures are above conventional dead burning temperatures. The double firing process is obviously energy intensive. But the pelletization process involved in between helps in uniformity of densification and growth in the doloma aggregates with improved and uniform properties. Since the impurity (like silica, alumina, iron oxide) present is low and the low melting liquid phases formed are less in amount, obtaining high densification is sometimes difficult in the dead burning process. Temperatures more than 1850°C are usually required to achieve satisfactory density and hydration resistance.

Generally high-grade dolomite, containing combined impurities less than 3%, is selected for dead burning. As it is difficult to densify high purity dolomite in a rotary kiln, it is customary to use some mineralizers to facilitate dead burning and get well dense aggregates. Iron oxide is a common additive for this purpose. The manufacturing process parameters vary with the grade of dead burnt dolomite to be produced. The dolomite after dead burning is cooled in either rotary or reciprocating recuperative coolers. When dead burning is done with an additive, it is necessary to use little higher firing temperature to shrink the dolomite in a reasonable time-cycle in the kiln.

Recently there are trends to use synthetic dolomite clinkers that contain no natural dolomite. Here calcium hydroxide is mixed with magnesium hydroxide with a small amount of additives, like iron oxide and fired at high temperature to get dead burnt dolomite clinker. The advantages of this type of aggregates are that the impurity phase present is completely controlled, and the composition can be adjusted as per the requirement of any particular application (CaO/MgO rich compositions). Hence, the properties can be tailored, and generally performance of the synthetic aggregates are better compared to natural ones, especially for the hot strength and corrosion resistance points of view.

Clinker/aggregates obtained by the dead burning process is crushed and ground to desired particle size level and mixed in proportions to obtain optimum packing. The fractions are first mixed in a mixer and then ~4% water is added for hydraulic pressing of the stabilized dolomite. Mix batch is then hydraulically pressed at 80–120 MPa and then dried. For water containing compositions, drying is critical as cracks may appear from hydration. To avoid any crack formation during drying, it is done with a stream of dry and clean air at temperatures below 60°C. To reduce the risk of hydration, in many a case water is avoided and wax is used as binder. To get a good flowability of wax and uniformity in the mixture little heating (~60°C) is done during the mixing process. The firing of dolomite refractories is done in both batch and continuous types of kilns. The temperature of firing the shapes depends on the chemical purity of the dolomite aggregate used. For high pure, dead burnt (not stabilized) dolomite firing is done more than 1700°C to get strong and well densified products.

Other than this conventional sintered dolomite refractories, there is tar/pitch bonded dolomite bricks used in steel making process. In this case dolomite is not calcined or dead burnt, raw dolomite is crushed, and ground and the different fractions are mixed with ~10% tar/pitch. Mixed compositions are then pressed hydraulically and tempered below 400°C. Due to low temperature processing, the cost of these types of refractories is low. Again presence of carbon (coming from the fixed carbon of tar/pitch) in these refractories helps in increasing the corrosion resistance.

9.4 CLASSIFICATIONS AND PROPERTIES

Dolomite refractories can be of different types as per the starting material used. It can be fully stabilized refractory which has relatively high silica (impurities) content, having strong hydration resistance but at the cost of formation of the liquid phase at lower temperatures and poor hot strength properties. Partially stabilized dolomite refractories are having lower extent of impurities and have only low temperature liquid coating at the surface resulting in strong hydration resistance and little improved hot properties compared to fully stabilized ones. Refractories with high temperature dead burnt dolomite clinkers with minimum impurities shows relatively better properties, but continuous attention and precaution are required to avoid hydration of the product.

Carbon bonded doloma refractories is also a special class that is economic and hydration resistant. These unfired dolomite refractories can be further subdivided according to the type of carbon binder used. Tar or pitch bonded unfired dolomite refractories are thermoplastic in nature, but resin bonded ones are thermosetting in character. Again pitch bonding graphitizes at higher temperatures resulting in better oxidation resistance compared to that of the "glassy natured carbon" from the resin bonded ones. But the resin bonded ones show higher strength values and lower fume emissions during preheating.

In general, properties of doloma refractories vary widely depending on the types of the aggregates used, their compositions and process of manufacturing. Doloma is made up of two very stable oxides and that too of high basic character. Hence, the refractory is very strong against molten steel and any basic slag. Generally, in contact with slag which is not saturated with the basic components, a layer of dense and highly viscous Ca/Mg silicate liquid forms due to the reaction between doloma refractory and slag components on the hot face of the refractory. Thus restricting the further slag corrosion and penetration and the overall corrosion resistance of the refractory is improved. Further improvement in the slag resistance of doloma refractories is done by addition of high purity magnesia in it. But if the slag is highly acidic in nature or contains lesser amount basic components compared to that of R_2O_3 components, low melting and low viscous liquids in the $CaO-Al_2O_3-Fe_2O_3-SiO_2$ system will form by dissolving the CaO or MgO of the refractory, thus resulting in high corrosion of the refractory. Also, doloma refractories are weak against slags containing high amount of iron oxide.

Softening of these refractories occur at very high temperatures, but the hot strength drastically deteriorates with the amount of impurity phase. Formation of low melting and low viscous Ca/Mg silicate phases are mainly responsible for lower strength properties at high temperatures. Good quality doloma has refractoriness (PCE) ~2300°C but RUL value ~1650–1700°C.

For doloma refractory, hydration resistance is important due to the presence of lime in it. Any free lime present in doloma reacts with atmospheric moisture and makes the material crumble on hydration. The degree of hydration is dependent on doloma refractory composition (amount of lime and impurities), densification, surface porosity, and time, temperature and relative humidity of the exposure to moisture. The degradation of doloma on hydration occurs in two stages

1. The formation of $Ca(OH)_2$ on the surface

2. Breaking apart of the refractory (grains) into smaller particles due to expansion

The hydration tendency is a major problem for the refractory manufacturers as the sintered grains cannot be stored for long. To control the hydration problem, attention and precaution at the critical stages of manufacturing of dead burnt aggregates and bricks are required. Immediate use of the freshly prepared doloma aggregates in the brick making also must be practiced, to reduce the risk of hydration with time. Better packaging techniques and equipment are to be used to retain the dehumidifying conditions for the fired bricks that can further control the crisis to a great extent. During application, the refractories are constantly at high temperatures and so chances of hydration (low temperature activity) is less.

Doloma is a solid solution of two oxides that are having relatively higher thermal conduction and thermal expansion properties among the different refractory oxides. Hence, it conducts higher amount of heat, may cause greater heat loss and moreover higher expansion properties cause degradation in the thermal shock properties. Again for fully or partially stabilized dolomites, type of silicate phase formed is important. The presence of di-calcium silicates (C_2S) is good due to its volume stability at high temperature, but phase inversion on cooling is a serious concern and requires proper attention. Again a significant improvement in the thermal shock resistance of doloma refractories was achieved by the addition of zirconia.

This is due to the microcracking effect caused by the formation of calcium zirconate phase (the formation is associated with volumetric expansion).

9.5 EFFECT OF IMPURITIES ON PHASE DIAGRAM

Doloma is a solid solution of CaO and MgO, and the details of the phase diagram are given in Figure 8.2. Both the oxides are individually high melting and have melting temperatures 2570°C and 2825°C, respectively. Though they satisfy most of the criteria to form a complete solid solution, a greater difference in their ionic sizes does not allow them to do so. They react and form a eutectic at 2370°C with a composition of 43.5% MgO and 56.5% CaO. But at room temperature, these oxides exist as a mixture.

Two component phase diagrams related to MgO are described in Chapter 8. Here the CaO related phase diagrams are discussed. The phase diagram of the $CaO–SiO_2$ system is also detailed in Chapter 8, Figure 8.1. The presence of silica in CaO reduces the liquidus temperature, and liquid phase starts forming at the peritectic temperature of ~2070°C, with a peritectic composition of ~25 mol% SiO_2. Generally, the naturally available doloma does not have silica more than this amount. So the presence of silica does not affect much on the liquid phase formation with CaO. But in a ternary system of $CaO–MgO–SiO_2$, the liquid phase may start even at a much lower temperature of ~1320°C close to diopside ($CaO \cdot MgO \cdot 2SiO_2$) composition.

Details of the phase diagram in the Ca–Fe–O system is given in Figure 9.1. The figure shows that both CaO and FeO can accommodate each other in their structure to a limited extent forming a partial solid solution, with a maximum limit at the peritectic temperature ~1100°C. But the effect of FeO on CaO is drastic, other than forming solid solution the formation of liquid phase starts even at the peritectic temperature, so when the amount of FeO exceeds the solid solution limit, liquid phase will exist even above 1100°C. However at low temperature FeO will exist as di-calcium ferrite ($Ca_2Fe_2O_5$) form. This only compound $Ca_2Fe_2O_5$ formed in the system decomposed to lime (CaO) solid solution and wustite (FeO) solid solution at ~1100°C.

Again the presence of Fe_2O_3 in CaO does not form any solid solution but drastically reduces the liquidus temperature to 1450°C which is the eutectic temperature between CaO and the compound di-calcium ferrite ($Ca_2Fe_2O_5$). Hence, this signifies that presence of any amount of Fe_2O_3 in CaO system will start producing liquid phase above 1450°C, and the amount of liquid will be dependent on the amount of Fe_2O_3 present.

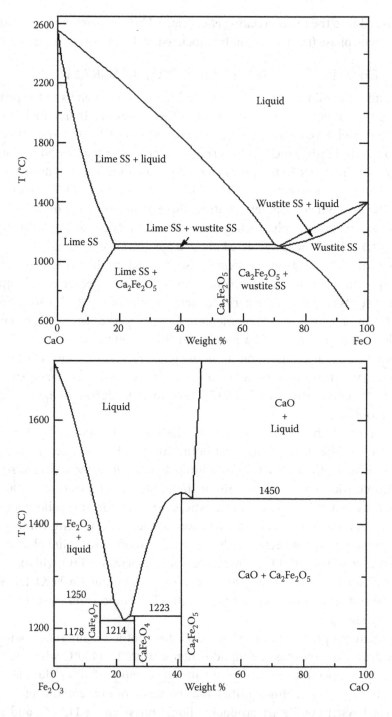

FIGURE 9.1   Phase diagram of lime (CaO) with FeO and Fe₂O₃.

9.6 MAIN APPLICATION AREAS

Dolomite refractories were widely used in steel making applications till say the 1980s, especially in the converter lining. But as the use of magnesia carbon has increased, the trend for using dolomite in converter has gone down abruptly. Dolomite was first used as refractory in the linings in open hearth furnaces or Thomas converters in 1878, where sodium silicate bonded dolomite stone was used and calcined *in situ* in the converter. Carbon bonded doloma was also important for the hearth application as the basic process of steel making gained ground and importance of removal of phosphorous and sulfur were recognized. During that days, much of the refractory were allowed to be consumed by the steel making process (CaO from dolomite refractory helps to from slag) and the doloma was not beneficiated and was also not highly pure.

With the increase in the lime addition as a flux in the converter, magnesia started replacing doloma due to higher refractory character and hydration resistance. Use of doloma refractory as a source of lime in the steel making process was no longer valid due to extra lime addition in the steel making batch composition. Carbon bonded doloma refractories were still continued. Even in 1980s, doloma were still competing with magnesia due to abundant availability and economy, mainly for LD converters and electric arc furnaces. But the availability of large grained magnesia and development of magnesia-carbon refractories has slowly removed the use of doloma refractories in primary steel making. But still it is important in secondary steel making processes even today.

For iron and steel industries, fired doloma refractories with 60% CaO and 40% MgO content are important for AOD (argon oxygen decarburization) converter and LRF (ladle refining furnace). Also, they are used in steel ladles. Again refractories with ~40% CaO and ~60% MgO are used for AOD and VOD (vacuum oxygen decarburization) converters. Pitch bonded doloma with 60% CaO and 40% MgO content are important for steel ladle and LRF applications whereas similar composition with resin bonding are useful for AOD, VOD, LRF, and steel ladle applications. Dolocarbon refractories, containing graphite in the compositions with resin bonding, are useful for the impact pads, slag lines, and other high wear areas in steel converters and steel ladles.

Use of dolomite refractories in burning zones of cement rotary kilns was started around the 1960s, mainly due to chemical compatibility with the cement manufacturing process and easy formation of a protective coating in the burning zone. The resistance of dolomite against alkalis is also important for cement kiln applications. ZrO_2 addition is also done in these bricks to improve the thermal shock resistance. Moreover, zirconia has a high refractoriness and is abrasion and corrosion resistant to clinker minerals. Zirconia containing doloma refractories have a high thermal elasticity and excellent thermal shock resistance. Formulations have also been developed using magnesia additions in dolomite to extend its use in the transition zones of the cement rotary kilns. Thus, chrome-free linings in the cement rotary kiln application was possible for environment friendly manufacturing.

For the cement making industry, 60% CaO and 40% MgO containing fired doloma refractories are important for the burning zones. For thermal shock prone areas of burning zones, ~58% CaO, ~38% MgO, and ~2% ZrO_2 containing compositions are used. High density, low porosity, less permeable brick with similar compositions are important for burning zones prone to chemical attack and gas penetration. Magnesia enriched doloma compositions (~48% CaO and ~48% MgO) with (~2%) or without ZrO_2 were important for the transition zones of cement kilns and burning zones with the unstable protective coating. Excess MgO in fine fraction helps to form a coat on free lime and insulate and protect it against the reaction with sulfur containing volatiles in the kiln atmosphere.

Dolomite is also important for repair mass and sometimes more suitable as a repair mass than shaped refractory due to its associated defects and disadvantages. About 60% CaO, 35% MgO, and ~4% Fe_2O_3 containing dolomite fettling mass is important for the wall and bottom repair of steel melting electric arc furnaces. Similar composition with lower Fe_2O_3 containing ramming mass is important for the back filling mass for AOD and LRF applications. Again ~58% MgO and ~33% CaO containing composition with gunning consistency is important for hot repair of steel converter, ladle, and electric arc furnaces. Also, ~55%–57% MgO and ~40% CaO containing compositions are important for cold repair of the hearth of electric arc furnace and AOD vessel.

Recently dolomite refractories have found a newer and technologically critical and important application, for producing clean steel. Aluminum killed steel manufacturers typically faces a crisis of alumina build up and clogging of the continuous casting refractories. Alumina clogging affects the life and performance of the refractories, reduces casting rate and productivity and deteriorates steel quality. This may occur in the ladle shroud, tundish nozzle, tundish slide gate plate bore, submerged entry shroud (SES), and submerged entry nozzle (SEN). Alloying elements like

Ti, Ce, La, etc. enhances the build up and enhances the crisis. Doloma based refractory composition (with high CaO content, ~60%) in the metal contact areas does not allow the formation of alumina build up due to the formation of low melting Ca-aluminate phases with the alumina depositions and prevents the clogging.

9.7 SUMMARY

Dolomite is a double carbonate of Ca and Mg and as a refractory doloma is used which is a solid solution of CaO and MgO.

Doloma, contains about 58% of CaO, is highly hygroscopic in nature, reacts with the moisture present in the atmosphere and forms Ca-hydroxide, associated with a volume expansion and causing cracking and shattering of the refractory shape.

In earlier days, intentionally low melting compounds were allowed to form to convert all the CaO to silicate based compounds and hydration tendency were prevented. These volume stable completely converted dolomites were termed as stabilized dolomite. But the presence of low melting compounds drastically deteriorated the high-temperature properties.

To improve the properties, only the surface of the doloma was allowed to coat with such low melting compounds, such products were termed as partially stabilized dolomite.

To avoid any incorporation of impurity phases and having hydration resistance, dolomite is fired at a very high temperature and used immediately for brick making after dead burning using non-aqueous binders. But after firing of the refractory shape, they need to be specially packed to avoid any contact with the atmospheric moisture.

Doloma refractories are very strong against any basic slag and mostly used for this advantage only. But other than hydration tendency, it has drawbacks like higher thermal expansion character and lower thermal shock resistances.

Doloma is mostly useful for the secondary steel making processes and mainly used for the lining of LRF, AOD, VOD, EAF, etc. Other than conventionally shaped refractory doloma is also important as repair mass, as fettling, ramming, gunning mass in all the different secondary steelmaking vessels. Also, doloma refractories are important for burning and transition zones of cement rotary kilns.

QUESTIONS AND ASSIGNMENTS

1. Describe the raw material dolomite.

2. Discuss the advantages and disadvantages of doloma refractories.

3. What is stabilization and why it is required for doloma?

4. What are the techniques used to restrict the hydration of doloma refractories?

5. What is the role of iron oxide in the stabilization of doloma refractories?

6. Discuss and compare the fully stabilized and partially stabilized doloma.

7. Describe the manufacturing technique of doloma refractories.

8. Detail the properties of doloma refractories.

9. Discuss the effect of impurities on doloma refractories.

10. Discus the main applications of doloma refractories.

11. What advanced application doloma can have?

BIBLIOGRAPHY

1. C. A. Schacht, *Refractories Handbook*, CRC Press, Boca Raton, FL, 2004.
2. A. R. Chesti, *Refractories: Manufacture, Properties and Applications*, Prentice-Hall of India, New Delhi, 1986.
3. J. H. Chesters, *Refractories—Production and Properties*, Woodhead Publishing Ltd., Cambridge, UK, 2006.
4. P. P. Budnikov, *The Technology of Ceramics and Refractories*, 4th edn., translated by E. Arnold, *Scripta Technica*, The MIT Press, Cambridge, MA, 2003.
5. Taikabutsu Gijutsu Kyōkai, *Refractories Handbook*, The Technical Association of Refractories, Tokyo, Japan, pp. 164–166, 1998.
6. Harbison Walker, *Handbook of Refractory Practice*, Harbison Walker Refractories Co., PA, pp. CR2–CR6, 2005.
7. *Dolomite for Metallurgical and Refractory Use—Specification*, Indian standard specification, IS-10346, 2004.
8. M. Rabah and E.M.M. Ewais, *Ceramics International*, 35, 813–819, 2009.
9. H. I. Moorkah and M.S. Abolarin, Investigation of the properties of locally available dolomite for refractory applications. *Nigerian Journal of Technology*, 24(1), 79–86, 2005.
10. *Product Catalog*, Resco Products, Inc., Pittsburgh, US, 2006.
11. M. Hillert, M. Selleby, and B. Sundman, An assessment of the Ca-Fe-O system. *Metallurgical Transactions A*, 21 (10), 2759–2776, 1990.
12. R. E. Johnson and A. Muan, Phase equilibria in the system CaO-MgO-iron oxide at 1500°C. *J. Am. Ceram. Soc.*, 48 (7), 359–364, 1965.

CHAPTER 10

Chromite and MgO–Cr$_2$O$_3$ Refractories (Chrome–Mag and Mag–Chrome)

10.1 INTRODUCTION

This chapter covers three different types of refractories, but all of them have a common component, chromite. Chromite is the principal ore of chromium in which the metal exists as a complex oxide (FeO·Cr$_2$O$_3$) form. Chromite is the only economically extractable natural source of chromium and in refractory, it is the source of desired component chromia (Cr$_2$O$_3$).

The usefulness of chromia as a refractory is based on its high melting point of 2180°C (3960°F), moderate thermal expansion, neutral chemical behavior, and relatively high corrosion resistance. Chromite enhances resistances against thermal shock and slag corrosion, volume stability, and mechanical strength of a refractory. In contact with ferric oxide (Fe$_2$O$_3$), it forms a complete solid solution (a homogeneous crystalline phase composed of Fe$_2$O$_3$ and Cr$_2$O$_3$ dissolved in one another) and in contact with ferrous oxide (FeO), it forms a iron chromate spinel and expands considerably, causing the shape to crumble (bursting).

Again, chromium is a transitional element and changes its valency with oxygen concentration (temperature) and results in different coloration. Also hexavalent chromium is a health hazard. Chromium has a higher diffusivity compared to other refractory oxides and diffuses out from the refractory and enters the other systems and colors it. Due to these issues, pure chromite refractory is relatively rare and it is used in combination with other oxides, mostly magnesia.

Refractory grade chromite requires high purity (the amount of combined Cr_2O_3 and Al_2O_3 should exceed 57%) with very low amount of silica. Other oxides present in chromite affects the refractoriness of the material and should also be within a limited range. The use of chromite in the refractory industries has decreased considerably over the last few decades mainly due to the changes in steelmaking technology and availability of more suitable refractories. However, it is still an important niche in the refractories industry for certain specific applications.

10.2 RAW MATERIALS AND SOURCES

The main raw materials used for making these three types of refractories are magnesia and chromite. We have already covered raw material sources of magnesia (in Section 8.2), so only details of chromite as a raw material is described in this chapter.

Chromium is found in a broad range of oxide and silicate minerals available in nature. Chromium (Cr) is the 13th most common element on the earth's crust with an average concentration of about 185 ppm. At standard temperature and pressure, chromium is a metal; it does not, however, occur in the native state. The most important chromium-bearing mineral is chromite, which is the only commercially viable ore of chromium. It has a spinel structure with the general formula of AB_2O_4, where A is a divalent and B is a trivalent metal ion.

Chromite ore predominantly contains the iron chromate spinel but is usually associated with the considerable amount of gangue materials, most commonly magnesium silicates. The naturally occurring chromite is a chromium-bearing mineral with a generalised formula of (Mg, Fe)O.(Cr, Al, Fe)$_2$O$_3$. Magnesium ion replaces the divalent iron and aluminum and ferric ions substitute the chromium ions. These substitutions can also be seen as mixing of different spinels, namely, iron chromate ($FeCr_2O_4$), magnesium chromate ($MgCr_2O_4$), magnesium aluminate ($MgAl_2O_4$), iron aluminate ($FeAl_2O_4$), etc. Other than these, the mineral may be associated with some silicates, which also increase the silica content in the mineral.

TABLE 10.1   Chemical Constituents (% by Mass) of
Different Chromite Ores Used in Refractory Industries

	Grade 1 % by Mass	Grade 2 % by Mass	Grade 3 % by Mass
Cr$_2$O$_3$	52 min	50 min	48 min
Total iron (as FeO)	16 max	16 max	16 max
MgO	15 max	15 max	15 max
SiO$_2$	3 max	7 max	9 max
Loss on ignition	1.5 max	1.5 max	1.5 max

Chromite commonly occurs in mafic and ultramafic rocks, which cover large portions of the earth's surface. Peridotite, an ultramafic rock dominated by olivine (magnesium iron silicate), is the common host for economic chromite mineral deposits. Peridotite contains on an average 1% to 2% chromite mineral as an accessory one. Most economic chromite mineral deposits contain concentrations of at least 25% chromite mineral.

Globally, chromite is available in a distributed manner, and the southern Ural area of Kazakhstan is the largest depositary of chromite. As per country-wise availability, the important resources are Kazakhstan, Zimbabwe, South Africa, Finland, India, and Brazil. About 15% of the total world chromite consumption is from the refractory industry. A typical analysis of a chromite suitable for the refractory purpose is 40%–55% Cr$_2$O$_3$, 12%–24% Al$_2$O$_3$, 14%–24% Fe$_2$O$_3$, 14%–18% MgO, and less than 10% SiO$_2$. As per the chemical constituents of the chrome ore, the ore can be graded into three categories, as detailed in Table 10.1. Grade 1 will result in the best quality of refractories.

10.3 BRIEF OF MANUFACTURING TECHNIQUES

10.3.1 Chromite Refractory

Hard and lumpy chromite ore is first crushed and ground to desired particles fractions and beneficiated by physical separation for the removal of dust and clayey materials. Commonly, tar is added as bonding material to bind the ore particles together. Little heating during mixing of tar is required for proper flowability of the mix in the presence of tar and better homogeneity. Water-based binders may also be used. The mixed composition is then generally pressed into shapes and dried slowly to avoid any crack generation. Firing can be done in batches or in continuous type of kilns, but slow firing is essential. Firing temperature varies between 1400°C and 1500°C depending on the impurities present.

Precautions are required during firing. Chemical reactions occur during firing due to the formation of different types of spinels among the oxide constituents present in it. Mainly the spinel formation (iron chromate) is associated with an expansion, which causes the expansion of the shape and bursting or shattering. This problem is termed as "cauliflower expansion" (under the microscope, the expansion appears to be like cauliflower). To accommodate the expansion in the stack of the refractories, the chromite bricks are stacked loosely inside the furnace with enough gap. Also to control and accommodate the expansion slowly within the refractory, they are fired slowly.

The addition of magnesia is done to control the cauliflower expansion and also for the formation of magnesium chromate spinel. Again magnesia helps to increase the low refractoriness of the gangue material (impurities) by forming magnesium-bearing compounds and improves the high-temperature properties of the refractories.

10.3.2 Chrome Magnesia Refractories

The fractions of magnesia and chromite ores are mixed to reach the desired composition of the refractory in an edge runner mill or a pug mill with a green binder. Mixed compositions are pressed by hydraulic pressing by applying a pressure of 80–100 MPa and then dried below 80°C to avoid any hydration cracks. Dried shapes are then fired in batch or continuous kilns between 1500°C and 1700°C depending on the compositions and the impurities present. Heating and cooling are done slowly to avoid any cracking. Here also, the precautions taken for pure chromite refractory are taken to accommodate any expansion that occurs during firing. There are also some unfired chemically bonded refractories that develop strength due to bonding materials present after drying and curing.

10.3.3 Magnesia Chrome Refractories

Magnesia and chromite are processed separately to get different fractions as required for the desired compaction and then mixed in the desired proportions to obtain the proper composition. Separate minerals or chemicals may be added during the mixing process to form a chemical bond within the refractory. Mixing is done with water and then dried slowly between 60°C and 80°C to avoid any hydration and hydration-related crack generation. Dried products are fired in batch or continuous types of kilns, and firing is done up to a maximum temperature of 1500–1700°C. To accommodate any expansion from any further spinel formation in the composition, firing is done in a controlled manner at a slow rate. Chemically bonded refractories are not fired but cured for strength development.

10.4 CLASSIFICATIONS AND PROPERTIES

10.4.1 Chromite Refractories

Demand and application of pure chromite refractories are very limited, and so there is nearly no subclasses of chromite refractories. The properties of chromite refractories depend on the amount and types of impurities and also on the control of the bursting character (due to expansion) during firing. In the chromite refractories, on firing, FeO present will oxidize to form Fe$_2$O$_3$. In reality, this causes an imbalance in divalent and trivalent cation ratio of original spinel structure of the chromite. The total amount of spinel will change as well. In the final fired products, two solid phases would appear: one is the spinel phase with MgO (and remaining FeO) and trivalent oxides (like Cr$_2$O$_3$, Fe$_2$O$_3$, etc.) and the second one consists of the solid solution of different trivalent oxides (like Cr$_2$O$_3$, Fe$_2$O$_3$, Al$_2$O$_3$, etc.).

As chromia is a heavy material, the bulk density of these refractories is high, and generally varies between 3.8 and 4.0 g/cm^3 with an apparent porosity between 24% and 28%. The refractoriness depends on the impurities present and is generally above 1900°C, and refractoriness under load varies between 1500°C and 1550°C. The presence of free silica in chromite is highly detrimental to its thermal shock resistance properties. Chromia is neutral in character. Hence, less impure chromite refractories show good resistance to chemical attack in different environments. They are resistant to basic slags (except reducing conditions) and fluxes. But the acidic slag and blast furnace slags slowly corrode the refractory.

10.4.2 MgO–Cr$_2$O$_3$ Refractories (Chrome–Mag and Mag–Chrome)

The major advancement in the technology of basic refractories started after about 1930s when fired composition of a combination of dead burnt magnesite and chromite showed improved character than that of the individual components. When a mixture of magnesia and chrome is fired, then the reduction in availability of divalent cation (due to oxidation of iron) is balanced by the free MgO present. MgO forms a spinel structure with the oxides of trivalent cations present in chromite and also with the newly formed Fe$_2$O$_3$. This MgO-containing spinels are high melting compounds and increases the application temperature of the composition with improved high-temperature properties. The spinels that may form in the MgO–Cr$_2$O$_3$ refractory compositions are FeCr$_2$O$_4$, MgCr$_2$O$_4$, FeAl$_2$O$_4$, and MgAl$_2$O$_4$. All these spinel phases are stable up to their high-temperature melting points. They are also congruent in character, which means that they do not decompose and melt to the liquid of its composition. Phase diagrams related to these spinel phases are given in Figure 10.1. Also, silica is a common impurity present in chromite ore, causing low melting silicate compounds. But the addition of free MgO also converts it to a high-melting forsterite (2MgO SiO$_2$) phase and the compositions have better high-temperature properties.

In MgO–Cr$_2$O$_3$ refractories, both in chrome–mag and mag–chrome types, the classification is done as per the bond phase present in the refractory. The

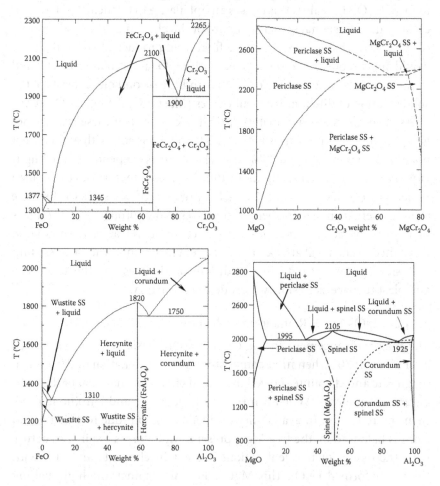

FIGURE 10.1 Phase diagram of different spinel compositions that may form in MgO–Cr$_2$O$_3$ refractories.

TABLE 10.2   MgO and Cr$_2$O$_3$ Content in
Different Types of MgO–Cr$_2$O$_3$ Refractories

Bonding	Magnesia Chrome	Chrome Magnesia
Chemical	MgO—55% min	MgO—30% min
	Cr$_2$O$_3$—6% min	Cr$_2$O$_3$—18% min
Sintering	MgO—75% min	MgO—50% min
	Cr$_2$O$_3$—6% min	Cr$_2$O$_3$—18% min

main bonding used in these refractories is the sintering bond or a chemical bond. The chemical compositions and properties of MgO–Cr$_2$O$_3$ refractories also change with the bonding system and the details of the amount of MgO and Cr$_2$O$_3$ variation with the bonding system is given in Table 10.2.

Chemical bonding is the simplest way to develop a bond in MgO–Cr$_2$O$_3$ refractories, which are basically unfired bricks. In chemical-bonded refractories, pressed shapes are dried and the bonding chemicals present (added during mixing), say phosphates and sulfates, harden due to chemical change or reaction with the refractory and provide strength. These chemically bonded MgO–Cr$_2$O$_3$ refractories have relatively lower hot strength and slag resistance and considered to be relatively economic with poor properties. As no firing is done, they can accommodate impure raw materials and usually used in low-cost compositions to balance out the wear profile in various application areas. But as the chemical bond degrades at an intermediate temperature, its strength deteriorates. In a modification to conventional chemical-bonded refractories, during pressing, some of the chemically bonded refractories are covered with steel plates, called metal-cased or steel-cased brick. Metal casing helps to retain the strength at intermediate temperatures and improves thermal shock resistance. Also, it helps to maintain the bond in the whole brick work during use, and as steel oxidizes at high temperatures, it bonds with one another and forms a tight bond between the whole brick structure. This type of refractories is useful for roof applications. However, the manufacturing and application of unfired MgO–Cr$_2$O$_3$ bricks are very limited.

Next to chemical bonding comes the fired MgO–Cr$_2$O$_3$ refractories. Initially, these refractories started with the firing of the mixture of dead burnt magnesia and chrome ore, which resulted in bonding and strength. But the presence of impurities, especially silica, resulted in a silicate bond within the refractory. A thin film of silica-based coating on magnesia and chrome particles provide strength. The firing of these refractories is dependent on the amount and types of impurities and silicate phases present in the system. Again due to the formation of low melting liquids at high temperatures from impurities and silicates, these refractories have low hot strength and corrosion resistances. Also presence of silicate-based glassy bond phase results in relatively lower thermal shock resistances. Though the development of fired $MgO-Cr_2O_3$ started with silicate bonding, it changed slowly to direct bonded refractories and presently used in very limited areas.

Reduction in or removal of impurity phases from the starting magnesia and chromite will minimize or remove the silicate phase present between the magnesia and chromite grains in the fired refractories. Hence, these magnesia and chromite grains will bond directly with each other to form the direct bonding. These directly bonded refractories are only possible by using high-purity raw materials and firing the pressed bodies to very high temperatures (>1700°C). The higher the temperature and longer the firing schedule, greater extent of reaction will take place, greater bonding will occur with a higher amount of spinel will be formed. Both the primary and secondary spinels will be found in the microstructure of the product, and the refractory will be volume stable and has high heat strength with great corrosion and thermal shock resistances. But obviously, these refractories are relatively costly compared to that of the chemically bonded or silicate-bonded ones.

There are also another variety of $MgO-Cr_2O_3$ refractories, which are termed as coburnt or rebonded refractory. In this case, high-purity raw materials (in fine form) are mixed as per desired proportions, pressed to pellet and coburnt (dead burning) in kilns (say rotary kiln) at very high temperatures. The resulting grains are dense and directly bonded in nature. These grains are used for making the shaped refractory by mixing in different fractions, pressing, and firing. As the expansion due to spinel formation has already occurred during coburning, these refractories shrink on firing and do not expand like the previous ones. These refractories are high volume stable, as nearly all the reactions (spinel formation) are completed in two different high-temperature firings, have the high hot strength and other high-temperature properties, and have much lower porosity, resulting in further improvement in corrosion resistance.

In a special variety of $MgO-Cr_2O_3$ refractories, fused magnesia–chrome grains are used to improve the corrosion resistance especially. Dead burnt magnesia and chrome ore are first mixed as per the desired proportions; then the mix is fused in an electric arc furnace, cooled, and then crushed and ground to get the desired fractions for making refractory shapes.

The shapes are then fired at high temperatures. As the reactions within the batch materials have already completed during fusion, these shapes also do not expand but shrink during the refractory firing. These refractories have lower porosity and fused grains, resulting in very high corrosion resistances and hot strength properties.

In general, properties of the MgO–Cr$_2$O$_3$ refractories depend on the composition, impurities present, and types of the bond present. Due to the presence of Cr$_2$O$_3$ in the compositions, all the refractories look gray to dark brown in color, depending on the amount of Cr$_2$O$_3$ and Fe$_2$O$_3$ present.

Refractoriness of these refractories are generally above 2000°C, and the RUL value is above 1700°C for the direct bonded, rebonded, and fused grained bricks. But due to the presence of the impurity phases and formation of the liquid phase at lower temperatures in chemically bonded and silicate bonded refractories, the RUL value is relatively low and varies between 1500°C and 1550°C.

Thermal spalling properties of MgO–Cr$_2$O$_3$ refractories vary with the amount of MgO and Cr$_2$O$_3$ content and the impurities present in the composition. Chrome–mag refractories have better spalling resistance than the individual magnesia or chrome refractories but have relatively lower thermal spalling resistance than magnesia–chrome refractories.

Regarding corrosion, refractories with chemical bonding and silicate bonding have poor resistance compared to that of the direct bonded, fused grains, and rebonded MgO–Cr$_2$O$_3$ refractories. The presence of impurities and formation of the liquid phase in the refractories strongly deteriorate the corrosion properties. Again when the compositions have higher Cr$_2$O$_3$ content, say in chrome–mag compositions, the refractories disintegrate in the presence of higher FeO in the slag. This may be the due absorption of FeO which causes expansion of the refractory. The more the amount of FeO, more is the absorption and the higher the degree of deterioration. Also the presence of CaO in the system (say in slag) further deteriorates the situation. Compared to chrome–mag refractories, mag–chrome refractories show a better performance against FeO corrosion. But at a very high concentration of FeO in slag or very high content of iron in chromite itself causes similar deterioration in the mag–chrome refractories. Hence among the different compositions of MgO–Cr$_2$O$_3$, high magnesia containing (say 80%) refractory is strong against a basic slag attack and alkali environment whereas a composition with a lesser amount of MgO (55%–60%) and high Cr$_2$O$_3$ (18%–25%) is stronger in the thermal spalling environment.

10.5 MAIN APPLICATION AREAS

Pure chromite refractories are available and used in a very limited manner. They are mostly used in reheating furnaces, like hearth of soaking pits and in rolling mills due to its high abrasion resistance. High Cr_2O_3 (95%) containing dense refractories are important for fiber glass furnaces in glass contact areas due to their excellent corrosion resistance. However, there are issues related to the coloring problem.

The use of $MgO-Cr_2O_3$ has started around 1930 and development continued till the end of the last century. They were most important for the basic open hearth furnaces and electric arc furnaces. But the application of these refractories has decreased greatly with the development and increased use of MgO–C refractories, reduction in steelmaking through open hearth furnaces, and use of water cooling for walls and roofs of electric arc furnaces. Still $MgO-Cr_2O_3$ refractories are important in many other applications, which are described as follows.

Magnesia–chrome refractories are commonly used in secondary steelmaking process due to the resistance against various basic slags and volume stability at high temperatures. Relatively low-grade mag–chromes are used as backup lining in the steel converter and steel ladle. Direct bonded and coburnt mag–chrome refractories are important for the degassing furnaces, like AOD and VOD, electric arc furnaces. As on today, degassers are the largest consumer of magnesia–chrome refractories. Coburnt mag chrome is useful for steel vacuum degasser. Chrome magnesite refractories are used for the sidewalls of the electric arc furnaces, soaking pits, and for the lining of induction furnaces. Electric arc furnaces (EAFs) used by the ministeel plants are conventionally lined with fused-cast mag–chrome refractories in the high-wear hot spots (walls nearest to the electrodes), direct bonded and coburnt mag–chrome in the remainder of the sidewalls and slag lines, and chemical-bonded and direct-bonded magnesia–chrome brick on the roofs. Stainless steel making EAFs also uses direct-bonded and rebonded fused-grain magnesia–chrome (60 wt% MgO) brick in the slag line and lower hot-spot areas of sidewalls.

Different copper making furnaces also use $MgO-Cr_2O_3$ refractories. The linings of copper converter and copper reverberatory furnaces are done with chrome–mag refractories. Again fused cast $MgO-Cr_2O_3$ composition is used in converter furnace bottom and tuyere zone, having the highest wear rate, to minimize corrosion. The tuyere area of copper converter has a higher rate of wear and generally lined with a better quality refractory compared to that of the rest of the converter. Like if silicate-bonded chrome–mag is used for the bulk lining, then direct-bonded mag–chrome is to be applied for the tuyere, but if direct-bonded refractory is used for the bulk of the wear lining, then rebonded, or fused-grain mag–chrome is to be used for tuyere areas.

Direct bonded high-temperature fired high MgO (80%–85%) containing mag–chrome refractories with little iron oxide are used in the burning and transition zones of cement rotary kilns due to their excellent strength, high volume stability, corrosion resistance, and easy coating formation.

Coburnt high-fired mag–chrome refractories are important for non-ferrous metallurgy like lead, zinc, and nickel furnaces due to their excellent corrosion, erosion, and thermal shock resistances.

10.6 HAZARDS WITH CHROMITE-CONTAINING REFRACTORY

It has been found by many research works that chromite-containing refractories form toxic compounds when they are exposed to high temperature, high pressure, and chemical contacts. Hexavalent chromium compounds, exceeding the United States Environmental Protection Agency (EPA) limits, were found in chrome-bearing materials when they are in contact with calcium aluminates. Prolong exposure to hexavalent chromium may cause lungs cancer (by breathing airborne Cr^{+6}), irritation and damage to the nose, throat, respiratory tract, eyes, skin, etc.

Environmentally hazardous hexavalent chromium containing CrO_3 forms in refractories along the grain boundaries. The transition of Cr^{3+} into Cr^{6+} in the air is accelerated when chromite is in contact with alkali and alkaline earth oxides. Hence, chromite-containing refractories must be avoided in contact with alkali and alkaline earth oxides, especially calcium oxide. The formation of Cr^{6+} may also be controlled by controlling the temperature, basicity (CaO/SiO_2), and chromite particle size used in making the refractory. The use of coarser chromite particles and fused grains resulted in a decreased formation of Cr^{6+} during refractory use.

Again, most of the refractories are disposed as landfill after use. Any conversion to Cr^{6+} will leach out in such disposal and is a great threat to the environment. Recycling, reuse, and waste management of the refractories are extremely difficult since these processes are associated with cost, difficulty in separation of contaminated part, and quantification of the quality product. Also, due to the risk of contamination, recyclable, spent refractories are low-value items and rarely get proper attention. A great thrust is required to recycle and reuse these chromite refractories, not only to protect the environment but also to make the process economic. Also, plenty of work has been done to substitute chromite-containing refractories in almost all the application areas, and many advanced countries have banned the use of Cr_2O_3-containing refractories as a safety measure.

10.7 SUMMARY

Chromite-containing refractories are mainly of three types, namely chromite, magnesia–chrome, and chrome–magnesia refractories.

Chromite is a natural mineral, ideally containing FeO and Cr_2O_3. But in natural occurrences, Fe is replaced mainly by Mg and Cr is replaced mainly by trivalent Fe and Al ions. Also, it is contaminated with silica. $MgO-Cr_2O_3$ refractories use magnesia, mainly in the pure dead burnt form and chromite as a natural raw material source.

Chromite refractories have nearly no classification. But $MgO-Cr_2O_3$ refractories are classified according to the content of Cr_2O_3 as mag–chrome and chrome–mag. $MgO-Cr_2O_3$ refractories are also classified on the basis of bonding, namely chemically bonded, silicate bonded, direct bonded, co-burnt or re-bonded, and fused grains types.

Chromite refractories and chemical bonded and silicate bonded $MgO-Cr_2O_3$ refractories have higher impurity content and have relatively poor heat properties and corrosion resistances. $MgO-Cr_2O_3$ refractories are mostly used in ferrous and non-ferrous metallurgical industries, cement kilns, and glass industries.

At high temperature, trivalent chromium may convert to a hexavalent state, which is a toxic material and presence of alkalis and calcium enhances the conversion. Hence, the use and disposal of chromium-containing refractories need special attention.

QUESTIONS AND ASSIGNMENTS

1. Discuss in detail about the chromite ore.

2. Write in detail about the manufacturing, properties, and applications of chromite refractories.

3. Discuss the different classifications of $MgO-Cr_2O_3$ refractories.

4. What are the different bonding systems used in $MgO-Cr_2O_3$ refractories? Discuss them.

5. Discuss the advantages and disadvantages of different bonding system in MgO–Cr$_2$O$_3$ refractories.

6. Discuss the difference in manufacturing techniques of different MgO–Cr$_2$O$_3$ refractories having different bonding.

7. Explain the applications of chromite refractories.

8. Discuss the applications MgO–Cr$_2$O$_3$ refractories.

9. What are the dangers of chromium-bearing refractories? Discuss.

BIBLIOGRAPHY

1. J. H. Chesters, *Refractories—Production and Properties*, Woodhead Publishing Ltd., Cambridge, UK, 2006.
2. P. P. Budnikov, *The Technology of Ceramics and Refractories*, 4th edn., translated by E. Arnold, *Scripta Technica*, The MIT Press, Cambridge, MA, 2003.
3. *Harbison-Walker Handbook of Refractory Practice*, Harbison-Walker, PA, 2005.
4. C. A. Schacht, *Refractories Handbook*, CRC Press, Boca Raton, FL, 2004.
5. A. Rashid Chesti, *Refractories: Manufacture, Properties and Applications*, Prentice-Hall of India, New Delhi, India, 1986.
6. W. David Kingery, H. K. Bowen, and D. R. Uhlmann, *Introduction to Ceramics*, 2nd edn., John Wiley and Sons Inc., New York, 1976.
7. Waing Waing Kay Khine Oo, Shwe Wut Hmon Aye, and Kay Thi Lwin, Study on the production of chromite refractory brick from local chromite ore. *World Academy of Science, Engineering and Technology*, 22, 569–574, 2008.
8. Waing Waing Kay Khine Oo, Shwe Wut Hmon Aye, and Kay Thi Lwin, Study on the production of chromite refractory brick from local chromite ore. *International Journal of Chemical, Molecular, Nuclear, Materials and Metallurgical Engineering*, 2(10), 234–239, 2008.
9. C. Kim, A. Kohler, K. Mulvaney, and L. Wagner, Chrome in refractories. *Ceramic Industry*, 142(8), 57–61, 1992.
10. A. Nishikawa, *Technology of Monolithic Refractories (Plibrico Company)*, p. 69, Toppan Printing Company, Japan, 1985.
11. D. J. Bray, Toxicity of chromium compounds formed in refractories. *American Ceramic Society Bulletin*, 64(7), 1012–1016, 1985.
12. C. G. Marvin, Chrome bearing hazardous waste. *American Ceramic Society Bulletin*, 72(6), 66–68, 1993.
13. L. B. Khoroshavin, V. A. Deryabin, V. A. Perepelitsyn, and T. N. Lapteva, Hexavalent chromium in refractories. *Ogneupory*, 9, 7–10, 1993.
14. J. P. Bennett and M. A. Maginnis, Recycling/disposal issues of refractories. *Ceramic Engineering and Science Proceedings*, 16(1), 127–141, 1995.

15. B. F. Belov, I. A. Novokhatskii, L. N. Rusakov, A. V. Gorokh, and A. A. Savinskaya, Phase diagram for an iron (II) oxide-chromium (III) oxide system. *Russian Journal of Physical Chemistry (Engl. Transl.)*, 42(7), 856–858, 1968.

16. A. M. Alper, R. N. McNally, R. C. Doman, and F. G. Keihn, Phase equilibria in the system MgO–MgCr$_2$O$_4$. *Journal of the American Ceramic Society*, 47(1), 30–33, 1964.

17. I. A. Novokhatskii, B. F. Belov, A. V. Gorokh, and A. A. Savinskaya, The phase diagram for the system ferrous oxide-alumina. *Russian Journal of Physical Chemistry (Engl. Transl.)*, 39(11), 1498–1499, 1965.

CHAPTER 11

Magnesia–Carbon Refractories

11.1 INTRODUCTION

Magnesia–carbon refractory is a composite type of unfired refractory essentially required for the steelmaking process. As the refractory contains carbon (graphite as a source), they are not fired, because carbon will oxidize at ambient firing conditions. Also carbon (graphite), being a hydrophobic material, does not disperse in water-containing system, so for proper and uniform distribution of carbon with magnesia, organic binders are used like pitch, tar, resin, etc., instead of water. These binders polymerize under certain conditions and retain the shape and provide strength. As on today, MgO–C refractories are essential for both the primary and secondary steelmaking processes.

The initial development and first use of basic refractories with carbon were started in the early 1950s. These early carbon-containing basic refractories resulted in only about 100 heats in converter. Poor repair technology and huge production pressure were also the reasons for reduced service life. Considerable improvement in the performance and life were obtained when magnesia fines were used in combination with the dolomite coarse fractions bonded with pitch. Further improvements came with all the magnesia pitch-bonded brick, replacing dolomite. Later, in 1970s, pitch-impregnated burnt magnesia bricks having reduced surface pore and pore size were developed for the charge pad and other high wear areas. This was the initiation of the zonal lining concept in basic oxygen furnaces. Slowly purity of magnesia became an important factor and highly pure (>96%) low boron-containing magnesia with lime:silica ratio above 2 became the preferred material.

After 1980s, slowly the conventional binders like pitch and tar were replaced by resin, mainly due to higher carbon (fixed) content and environmental friendliness. Use of additives like antioxidants also started to improve the performance and service life. High-quality magnesia and carbon with specific characteristics are being used to improve the corrosion resistance and other heat properties further.

At present, the MgO–C refractories are prepared by using high-quality magnesia and carbon sources and bonded with high carbon containing organic binder (say resin), with some metallic powder as antioxidants to protect the carbon. These MgO–C refractories are shaped at high pressure and are tempered or cured but not fired. The main features of MgO–C refractories are as follows:

1. High refractoriness as no low melting eutectic occurs between MgO and C.

2. Graphite, the carbon source, has very low thermal expansion; hence, the composite has also a low expansion value.

3. Graphite, having a unshared free electron, has very high thermal conductivity, which imparts high thermal conductivity in the MgO–C composite.

4. As the thermal expansion is low and the thermal conductivity is high, the thermal shock resistance of MgO–C refractories is very high.

5. As carbon molecules have very strong covalent bonding, they do not react much and do not get wet by any liquid. This non-wetting character results in very high corrosion resistance in MgO–C refractories against molten metal or slag.

6. Graphite has a low modulus of elasticity, hence has the ability to absorb stress with minimum deformation, thus keeping down the amount of discontinuous wear due to cracks.

Conceptually, the presence of carbon in magnesia refractory can be termed as magnesia–carbon (MgO–C) refractory. So in this broad description, carbon-containing magnesia refractories are of three types:

- Sintered and impregnated (pitch/tar) magnesia, containing up to 3% carbon.

- Tar/pitch bonded magnesia, containing up to 7% carbon.

- Carbon (graphite) containing magnesia, containing carbon about 8%–30%.

But conventionally, the third category of refractories is considered as MgO–C refractories and being considered all over the world.

11.2 RAW MATERIALS, BINDERS, AND ADDITIVES

Magnesia–carbon refractories are made up of two major components, namely magnesia and carbon. Other than these, antioxidants are used as additives, and an organic binder is required for shaping and providing strength after curing or tempering.

11.2.1 Magnesia

Magnesia constitutes the major portion of magnesia–carbon refractory, varying between 80% and 90% by weight. Three different types of magnesia are used for magnesia–carbon refractories, namely, fused magnesia, produced by fusing magnesia in an electric furnace, seawater magnesia produced by very high-temperature firing of magnesium hydroxide extracted from seawater, and sintered magnesia produced from natural magnesite. Details of the magnesia raw materials are discussed in Section 8.2. Being the major part, magnesia plays the pivotal role in the property development and performance of the MgO–C refractory. There are different selection criteria for magnesia to improve the quality of the refractory. These criteria are

1. High purity

2. High ratio of CaO/SiO_2

3. Minimum content of B_2O_3

4. Large periclase crystal size to reduce the grain boundary area

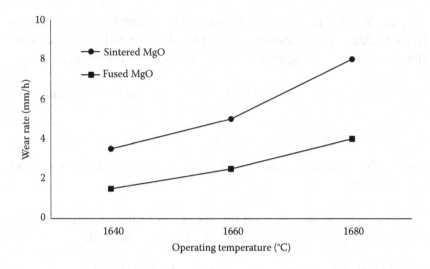

FIGURE 11.1   Effect of fused and sintered magnesia grains on the wear rate (corrosion) of the MgO–C refractory.

Use of impure magnesia will produce low-melting phases in the system, degrading the hot strength and corrosion properties against molten metal and slag. The similar effect will also be present if magnesia with lower lime:silica ratio or higher B_2O_3 content is taken. The use of fused grains results in increased periclase crystal sizes and provides higher corrosion resistances. Figure 11.1 shows the effect of fused and sintered magnesia grains on the wear rate (corrosion) of the MgO–C refractory. Increased temperature enhances the rate of corrosion due to higher slag fluidity. Fused magnesia containing refractory showed much higher corrosion resistance than the sintered ones. But larger crystals may affect the mechanical and thermal shock resistance properties, due to reduced number of grain boundaries and less resistance to crack propagation. So a mixture of fused and sintered magnesia is used, and the proportion is optimized as per the specific application area requirement.

11.2.2 Graphite

Carbon plays very vital role in MgO–C refractories due to its non-wetting character. But carbon has the instantaneous oxidation tendency at high temperatures in oxidizing atmosphere, generally prevailing in the user industries. Oxidized MgO–C refractory has a porous structure, with very low strength and corroding liquids can enter in it, resulting in a drastic deterioration of the refractory quality. Among different commercial sources of carbon, graphite shows the highest oxidation resistance. So it is selected as a carbon source in MgO–C refractories. Again as the flaky nature imparts higher thermal conductivity and lower thermal expansion, resulting in very high thermal shock resistance, flaky graphite is the preferable material as a carbon source.

Impurities present in graphite adversely affect the corrosion resistance of MgO–C brick. As flaky graphite is a natural mineral, it is often contaminated with quartz, muscovite, pyrite, feldspar, iron oxide, and kaolinite. These impurities produce ash after oxidation of graphite and decrease high-temperature properties and corrosion resistance of MgO–C refractory. These impurities may react with MgO or with the slag component in contact and form low-melting compounds, degrading the corrosion resistance of the refractory sharply. Hence, impurities and ash content of graphite should be as low as possible, and purity should be very high.

The role of graphite in MgO–C refractories are as follows:

1. Graphite, being a fine material fills the space between magnesia grains and produces compact structure.

2. The non-wetting character of graphite provides very high resistance to metal and slag corrosion and penetration into the refractory.

3. Due to high thermal conductivity and low thermal expansion, it improves the thermal spalling resistance.

11.2.3 Antioxidants

Oxidation of carbon is the main drawback of carbon-containing refractories. The oxidation of carbon in MgO–C refractories may occur in two ways: (a) direct oxidation and (b) indirect oxidation. Direct oxidation occurs below 1400°C when carbon is oxidized directly by the oxygen from the atmosphere.

$$2C(s) + O_2(g) = 2CO(g)$$

Indirect oxidation occurs generally above 1400°C where carbon is oxidized by the oxygen from MgO or slag (mainly FeO). The resulting Mg gas is discharged to the surface of the refractory along with CO(g) through the porous structure and gets oxidized to form MgO (secondary oxide phase). This nascent MgO gets deposited on the hot face of the refractory, and forms a dense layer that acts as an oxide coating and prevents further oxidation.

$$C(s) + MgO(S) = Mg(g) + CO(g)$$

$$C(s) + FeO(l) = Fe(l) + CO(g)$$

$$2Mg(g) + O_2(g) = 2MgO(s)$$

But in both the cases, carbon gets oxidized, and refractory becomes porous, weak in strength, and gets corroded easily. To prevent the oxidation of carbon, antioxidants are used. Antioxidants are materials that get oxidized faster by reacting with an incoming oxygen and protects the carbon from oxidation. These materials are simple metal powders that oxidize faster and easily. Generally, powders of magnesium (Mg), aluminum (Al), silicon (Si) metals, or fine boron carbide (B_4C) and silicon carbide (SiC) are used as antioxidants. Due to the low cost and high effective protection, Al and Si metal powders are mostly used, which after oxidation form respective oxides, remain as a stable discrete phase in the refractory, even at high temperatures.

$$4Al(s) + 3O_2(g) = 2Al_2O_3(s)$$

$$2Mg(s) + O_2(g) = 2MgO(s)$$

$$Si(s) + O_2(g) = SiO_2(s)$$

During operation at high temperatures, carbon also reacts with the metal powders forming metal carbides. For example, for Al-containing compositions, Al_4C_3 is formed. This reaction provides extra bonding to the refractory, resulting in further improvement of strength. Al metal powder melts around 660°C, which then reacts with carbon and forms the carbide.

$$4Al(l) + 3C(s) = Al_4C_3(s)$$

This carbide formation is especially effective in increasing the hot strength of the MgO–C refractory. Figure 11.2 shows that metal additives

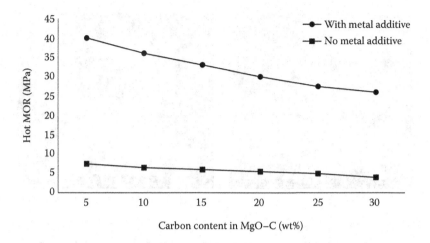

FIGURE 11.2 Variation of hot strength values of MgO–C refractory with and without metal additives against carbon content.

enhance the hot strength considerably compared to compositions without metal additives. The fall in strength in both the cases with increasing carbon content is due to enhanced oxidation of carbon in the composition, resulting in a more porous structure. Again for Al metal powder containing compositions, the formed Al_2O_3 reacts with MgO fines present in the matrix phase and forms the $MgO \cdot Al_2O_3$ spinel. This spinel formation is associated with a volume expansion that occurs within the refractory. This increased volume fills up the pores and reduces porosity. This also helps in reduction of the oxidation and corrosion of the refractory.

$$4Al(s) + 3O_2(g) = 2Al_2O_3(s)$$

$$Al_4C_3(s) + 6CO(g) = 2Al_2O_3(s) + 9C(s)$$

$$Al_2O_3(s) + MgO(s) = MgO \cdot Al_2O_3(s)$$

The formation of aluminum carbide and spinel phases is also observed in the matrix part of MgO–C refractories, as shown in Figure 11.3. Phase analysis also indicates and confirms the formation of these phases, but the intensity of these phases is relatively low due to the very little extent of the formation.

As an antioxidant, Al metal powder is preferred and widely used as it effectively prevents the oxidation, provides enhanced hot strength at

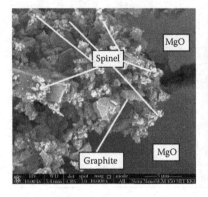
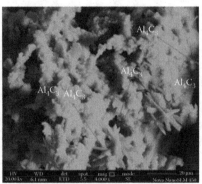

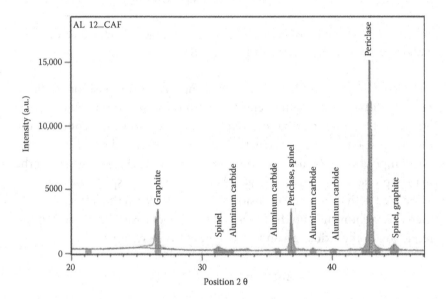

FIGURE 11.3 Formation of aluminum carbide and spinel phases in the microstructure and phase analysis of MgO–C refractories.

relatively low cost. However, MgO–C refractory with Al metal powder as an antioxidant suffers from some shortcomings. At low temperatures, the formed carbide phase (Al_4C_3) reacts with the water vapor and expands enormously, forming crack and reducing the service life. The formation of voluminous $Al(OH)_3$ and CH_4 (methane) gas causes the expansion and disintegration of the refractory.

$$Al_4C_3(s) + 12H_2O(g) = 3CH_4(g) + 4Al(OH)_3(s)$$

This is especially important for refractory linings when they are cooled to ambient temperature for intermittent repairs, which may take several days. In rainy seasons, humidity is high, and this may cause serious damage or deterioration of the whole refractory lining due to this hydration of the carbide phase.

Boron carbide behaves in a different manner as an antioxidant. It reacts with oxygen or CO and forms B_2O_3. This B_2O_3 is a low melting material and as a liquid, it coats the carbon particles. Also, it reacts with MgO and form low melting liquid phase compound $MgO \cdot B_2O_3$:

$$2B_4C(s) + 6O_2(g) = 4B_2O_3(l) + 2C(s)$$

$$B_4C(s) + 6CO(g) = B_2O_3(l) + 7C(s)$$

$$B_2O_3(l) + 3MgO(s) = Mg_3B_2O_6(s)$$

The melting point of $Mg_3B_2O_6$ is 1360°C, and liquid $Mg_3B_2O_6$ fills up the pores. It also acts as a good oxygen barrier above its melting point as it forms a thin coating on the brick surface that restricts the oxygen diffusion into the refractory. Thus, B_4C protects the carbon of MgO–C bricks in a better way against oxidation. But the amount of B_4C used has to be judiciously judged and any excess amount will produce greater extent of the liquid phase and will degrade the high-temperature properties of the refractory drastically. The addition of SiC also forms the SiO_2 layer and prevents oxidations and an excessive amount of silica is detrimental for MgO–C refractories.

11.2.4 Resin

It has been already mentioned that water cannot be used for mixing of carbon-containing compositions, so organic liquids are used. Again, the graphite used has a flaky structure and so it has very poor compressibility. That is, when the pressure is released after shaping or after drying process, graphite will spring back to its original dimensions if it is not held tightly and the refractory will expand. Hence, very strong binder is required for MgO–C refractories that can strongly hold the graphite flakes together (as in under pressed condition) after pressing and retain the pressed shape and dimensions.

The development of magnesia–carbon refractories started with impregnation of liquid pitch and tar in sintered dolomite or magnesia refractories.

This impregnation imparts a coating of carbon on oxide refractory and improved the corrosion resistance. These carbonaceous materials, tar or pitch, were first tried as organic binder. But during curing or tempering stage (for carbon–carbon network formation and development of strength) of the tar- and pitch-bonded refractories, huge amount of toxic fumes, containing polycyclic aromatic hydrocarbons (PAH) such as benzo-alpha pyrenes (BAP) (carcinogenic material), etc. are liberated. Later use of phenolic resin has started as bond material replacing tar and pitch. The advantages of phenolic resin are as follows:

- Greater chemical affinity to graphite, so easy dispersion

- Highly adhesive in nature resulting in dense shape with good strength

- A lesser extent of toxic gas evolution

- Excellent kneading and pressing properties

- Higher amount of fixed carbon

- Liberates mainly phenol and not PAH compounds during tempering

Phenolic resins are of two types: thermosetting (resol) and thermoplastic (novolac). Thermosetting resins give greater dried strength and high resistance against lamination (lamination occurs due to the presence of flaky graphite). Again thermoplastic resins require a chemical to set or harden, called hardener (like hexamine), and they provide greater mix life (conservation of mix quality for a longer time before mixing). Polymerization of the resin occurs due to tempering at around 200°C and leads to an isotropic interlocking structure that holds the refractory composition in three dimensions and provides strength. However, the resins have the limitation regarding their cost in comparison with pitches.

Viscosity (fluidity) of resol resin varies with temperature, and so it behaves differently in different seasons, like winter and summer. Heating may be required during mixing to obtain the proper dispersion of fines (including graphite) in winter and again in summer, the green body becomes soft due low viscosity, resulting in lamination. To overcome such crisis, powder novolac resin is mixed with the liquid resol resin. The increase in resin content improves the compressibility during pressing and corresponding strength of the tempered samples.

11.3 BRIEF OF MANUFACTURING TECHNIQUES

The manufacturing of MgO–C refractories involve no firing or sintering, but the refractory has to get similar kind of compaction and strength as they are mostly used in most critical areas of steel manufacturing. Hence, the critical stages of manufacturing these refractories are pressing, where initial compaction is given, and curing or tempering, where the bond material polymerizes to form a three-dimensional carbon chain network providing strength to the refractory even at high temperatures.

In the manufacturing process, first the raw materials, namely, sintered and fused magnesia of different size fractions, graphite, and additives (mainly antioxidant) are mixed and during mixing organic binder (resin) is added. Mixing continues for about 30 min, if required heating may be done depending on the resin viscosity. Resin viscosity in the range of 6000–8000 cps is maintained for proper distribution of graphite and other fines. Proper mixer is also required for better mixing performance as some kneading action is also necessary for better homogeneity in the batch. Generally, small-capacity heavy-duty mixers are used to get proper mix quality with a uniform coating of binder on the aggregate particles. After mixing, the mixture is allowed to age for a few hours, which helps for the polymerization of carbon to take place by the carbon–carbon interlocking mechanism. The controlled atmosphere (to maintain temperature and, humidity, etc.) aging is also done in some cases. The aged mixture is then shaped, generally by uniaxial pressing in a hydraulic or friction press. The presses should be enabled with the deairing system to remove the entrapped air from the batch mixture (to reduce or remove lamination) and capable of very high pressure generation. The durability and performance of MgO–C refractories depend on the compaction, density, and porosity of the body, so a very high pressure, up to about 200 MPa, is used for compaction. After pressing, the shapes are tempered or cured. Tempering or curing is the heat treatment process at low temperature to remove volatile matters from the organic binders and formation of carbon chain network that imparts strength. Tempering is done between 180°C and 250°C depending on the type and properties of the resin. Flow diagram for the manufacturing process is outlined in Figure 11.4.

11.4 CLASSIFICATIONS AND PROPERTIES

The classification of MgO–C refractories is based on the composition of the refractory, mainly the carbon content. The properties and performance of the refractory change with the amount of carbon and their application

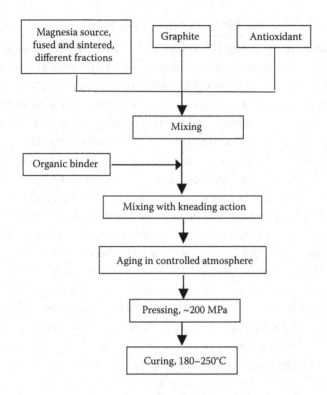

FIGURE 11.4   Flow diagram for manufacturing of MgO–C refractory.

areas too. An increasing amount of carbon will reduce the bulk density as lighter graphite will be replacing denser magnesia in the batch. In parallel, it will also reduce strength as it hinders any direct bonding between magnesia particles and also the elastic modulus, as graphite is a soft material (lower modulus of elasticity). Again the oxidation of the refractory will increase. But increasing carbon means higher thermal conductivity and lower thermal expansion of the composition, which result in greater thermal shock resistance. Also, corrosion and penetration resistances will significantly increase due to the non-wetting character of graphite.

Hence, an optimization in the carbon content is essentially required to get ideal properties for a specific application. It has been observed, as shown in Figure 11.5, that increasing amount of carbon content reduces the corrosion of the refractory, represented as corrosion index, where corrosion of the without carbon-containing composition is taken as 100. But over 20% of carbon content in the refractory leads to an enhancement of corrosion. An increasing amount of carbon enhances the non-wetting character in the composition and reduces the corrosion effectively. But oxidation of the

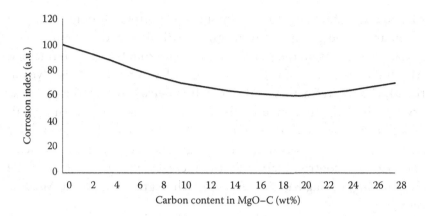

FIGURE 11.5   Effect of carbon content on the performance of MgO–C refractory.

refractory also increases, which produces a porous structure. At the lower amount of carbon, oxidation is less so effective resistance against corrosion, which increases with increasing carbon content. But at a higher level, oxidation is also strong and the benefit of non-wetting character due to the presence of higher carbon is nullified by oxidation of carbon. A minimum corrosion is observed for the composition containing about 20% carbon.

Though these refractories are not fired, they are very dense due to high pressing, and bulk density varies between 2.8 and 3.1 g/cc depending on the carbon content and has low apparent porosity, in the range of 4%–6%. Cold strength and hot strength (HMOR) also varies from about 60 to 18 MPa for 8% carbon batches to 30 and 10 MPa for the 20% carbon containing composition, respectively.

11.5 DEGRADATION OF MgO–C REFRACTORIES

MgO–C refractories are composite in nature and have the benefits of both the components. They are applied in very stringent and critical environments of steelmaking process. MgO–C refractories are essential in a few applications, and there is no substitute for them regarding the performance and service life in such critical applications. But still, they degrade due to many reasons. The main reasons for the degradation of MgO–C refractories are detailed below.

11.5.1 Dissolution of Magnesium by Slag

If the slag is low in basicity, then it will react with the basic MgO and SiO_2 present in the slag, leading to the formation of magnesium-containing silicates. This dissolution of magnesia will continue through the grain boundaries, and grain size of magnesia will decrease in contact with silicate slags. Finally, the grain will dislodge from the main refractory. Also higher presence of FeO in the slag will also react and dissolve out the MgO from refractory and slag will penetrate within the periclase crystals. In real situation, both the dissolution mechanisms run parallel and cause degradation of refractory very strongly. The use of purer MgO particles with larger size (fused grains) reduces these problems and also slag control, mainly by the increase in MgO content of the slag and higher slag basicity restricts such degradation of the MgO–C refractory.

11.5.2 Oxidation of Carbon

The oxidation of carbon produces a void space in the refractory; the porous structure of refractory is weak in strength, the non-wetting character falls drastically, and easily penetrated by corrosive liquids. Oxidation may occur in the liquid phase and in the slag, where oxidizing components of slag oxidize the carbon. Slag oxidation occurs mainly due to the presence of FeO. An increasing amount of iron in slag drastically degrades the quality of the refractory and causes high wear. The presence of manganese oxide also increases the wear rate.

Oxidation of MgO–C refractory by gaseous components is mainly due to oxygen and carbon dioxide. The gaseous oxidation is strong when the hot refractories are exposed to open atmosphere and in contact with gases. Gases directly react with the carbon and form its oxides. During the charging and discharging of molten metal and inspection or repair stage of refractories, refractories are highly susceptible to gaseous oxidation. The introduction of slag splashing technique after metal tapping (from converter) in steelmaking process helps to prevent such oxidation. Slag splashing helps to coat the refractory by a thin layer of liquid slag and hinders the gaseous components to come in contact with the refractory. But when slag-coated refractory is cooled (mainly during repair) below the slag melting temperature (~1000°C), the slag coating will solidify and shrink, causing crack and peeling of the coat and exposing the refractory to open atmosphere. Thus causes a sudden and huge oxidation. Figure 11.6 shows the beneficial effect of slag splashing and the effect of cooling of the MgO–C refractory on the oxidation behavior of the MgO–C refractory.

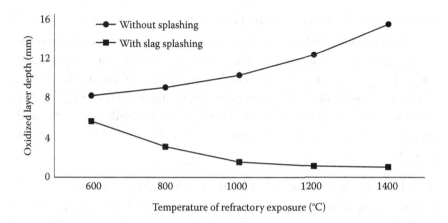

FIGURE 11.6 Effect of slag splashing in steel converter on the oxidized layer depth of MgO–C refractory.

Carbon also gets oxidized by magnesia. Though MgO–C refractory is considered as a composite refractory, still there is some reaction between these components at high temperatures. Magnesia reacts with carbon and gets reduced to pure magnesium and carbon converts to its oxides. This reaction may occur even within the refractory interior at high temperatures, and the product gases come out to the surface through the pores and a porous structure is generated by this oxidation. Magnesium vapor on the surface of the refractory reacts with the available oxygen from the atmosphere and converts to magnesia again. Thus, a newly formed magnesia layer covers the hot face of the refractory, reduces the surface porosity, and thus prevents further oxidation and also penetration of slag.

$$MgO(s) + C(s) = Mg(g) + CO(g)$$

$$Mg(g) + \frac{1}{2}O_2 = MgO(s)$$

However, the structure of the refractory will become porous and will result in degraded properties. This MgO and C reaction can be controlled by increasing the crystal size of the MgO grain, by using less reactive fused MgO and also by reducing the impurities of magnesia and increasing the lime:silica ratio.

11.5.3 Abrasion by Molten Steel and Slag

Degradation of the refractory also caused by the abrasion of the molten steel, especially in those areas where molten metal and slag has greater movement or impact. Physical wear due to mechanical action along with chemical dissolution due to the presence of moving fresh slag are the main reasons for this degradation. This can be controlled by dense and strong refractories, use of metallic additives, and lower carbon-containing refractories.

11.5.4 Degradation Due to Thermal and Mechanical Spalling

MgO–C refractories are susceptible to thermal and mechanical wear due to the stringent application conditions. Use of strong and dense refractories with proper carbon content and proper design and arrangement of refractories are required to reduce this type degradation.

11.6 MAIN APPLICATION AREAS

MgO–C refractories are only used in steel manufacturing process and to be specific, mainly in the steelmaking basic oxygen furnace (BOF) converters, steel ladles, and electric arc furnaces (EAF). Figure 11.7 shows the different areas of converter and ladle where MgO–C refractories are used. The major differences in quality of refractory used in the different application areas are their composition and associated properties.

For BOF working lining, mainly affected by slag and metal corrosion, MgO–C refractory with about 18% carbon is used. Higher carbon reduces the strength but for such applications, corrosion is most important and not the strength. But strength is important for the charge pad of BOF where the liquid metal and all other steelmaking batch materials fall from a height. An MgO–C refractory with about 9%–10% carbon is used for the charge pad and bottom applications. Once the charging is completed, these refractories will be covered under molten metal bath and hardly there will be any slag corrosion. So to resist the impact of falling batch materials, low carbon high strength MgO–C refractories are used. Low carbon results in relatively lower corrosion resistances of these refractories, but in the bottom application, the refractory is completely covered with liquid metal, and attack from slag is rare, so corrosion resistance is not of prime importance for the bottom. The whole BOF is hanging through metallic supports and effect of stresses due to the hanging condition exists in the trunnion area. Also, the stresses increase due movement of the BOF during steelmaking

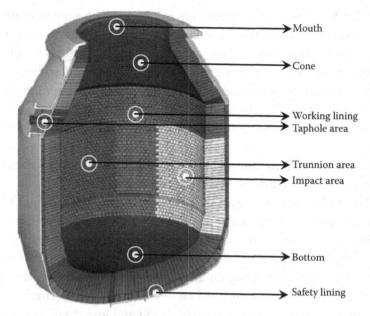

Steelmaking converter

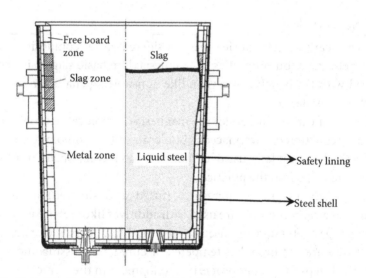

Steel ladle (left side before use and right side after use, corrosion)

FIGURE 11.7   Details of steel converter and steel ladle for application of MgO–C refractory.

process. So refractories in these areas require strength along with flexibility and about 12%–15% carbon containing MgO–C compositions are used for such applications. Similarly for taphole area, the refractories are under the tremendous movement of molten metal during tapping, so both the corrosion and strength are important in these areas and strong refractories containing about 12%–13% carbon are used for these applications.

For EAF slag zone, hot-spot and taphole areas, MgO–C refractories with 10%–12% C are used. Also, relatively strong refractories containing about 8% carbon are important for EAF and for secondary steelmaking like VOD and vacuum arc degassing (VAD) processes.

For steel ladle slag zone areas, MgO–C refractories with about 12% carbon are used whereas for the metal zone, as the corrosion effect is much reduced, refractories containing about 6%–8% carbon are used. Again in the ladle bottom, where high strength is required for the impact of metal fall, refractories containing about 5% carbon are used. But for the top part of the ladle (free board zone) where the temperature, strength, and corrosion are not so critical, low-carbon (5%) and low-strength refractories are used.

11.7 SUMMARY

Magnesia–carbon refractories are considered as a composite refractory where the good properties of magnesia, like basic slag resistance, is clubbed with the benefits of carbon like non-wetting character and thermal shock resistances.

The use of carbon in developing magnesia–carbon refractories started with impregnation of carbonaceous binder in sintered dolomite and magnesia refractory and later use of carbon as a batch component in the form of graphite came into the practice.

High-purity magnesia aggregates (fused and sintered) along with graphite as a carbon source are used with additives like metal powders and resin as organic binders are used in making MgO–C refractories. These refractories are not fired, but tempered or cured, so pressing and curing are critical steps for proper property development in the refractory.

An increase in carbon content enhances the non-wetting character and thermal shock resistances but also increases the chances of oxidation, resulting in a porous and weak structure, easily corroded, and penetrated by slag. A maximum of 20 wt% carbon is optimum for the performance of the refractory.

The degradation of MgO–C refractory occurs due to different factors during use, like dissolution of magnesia in slag, oxidation of carbon, abrasion of molten metal and slag, and mechanical and thermal spalling.

These refractories are mainly used in steelmaking converter (BOF), EAF, steel ladles, and secondary steelmaking. The complete BOF lining is done by these refractories with varying carbon content, due to stringent application conditions.

QUESTIONS AND ASSIGNMENTS

1. Why is carbon used in combination with magnesia?

2. Describe the selection criteria for magnesia and carbon for manufacturing MgO–C refractories.

3. What is an antioxidant? Describe its role in the performance of MgO–C refractory.

4. Discuss the advantages and disadvantages of different antioxidants used in MgO–C refractory.

5. Why is organic binder used in MgO–C refractory? Why is resin a preferred binder?

6. Briefly describe the manufacturing technique of MgO–C refractory.

7. Describe the effect of increasing carbon content in MgO–C refractory?

8. What is the maximum carbon amount used in MgO–C refractory and why?

9. Describe in detail the how MgO–C refractories degrade.

10. Describe the different ways of oxidation of carbon in MgO–C refractory.

11. Describe the applications of MgO–C refractories.

12. Describe in detail with the reasoning for the use of different MgO–C refractories in steel converters.

13. Describe how one can improve the oxidation behavior of MgO–C refractory.

BIBLIOGRAPHY

1. *Refractories Handbook*, The Technical Association of Refractories, Tokyo, Japan, 1998.
2. Harbison Walker, *Handbook of Refractory Practice*, Harbison Walker Refractories Co., PA, 2005.
3. C. G. Aneziris, J. Hubalkova, and R. Barabas, Microstructure evaluation of MgO–C refractories with TiO 2- and Al-additions, *Journal of the European Ceramic Society*, 27(1), 73–78, 2007.
4. U. Klippel and C. G. Aneziris, Prospects of ceramic nanoparticles as additives for carbon-bonded MgO–C refractories, *Proceedings of the 49th International Colloquium on Refractories*, Aachen, Germany, pp. 6–9, November 7–8, 2006.
5. C. G. Aneziris and U. Klippel, Thermal shock behaviour of carbon bonded MgO–C refractories with inorganic micro- and nano-additions, *CFI/Ber. DKG*, 83 (10), E50–E52, 2006.
6. C. G. Aneziris, U. Klippel, W. Schärfl, V. Stein, and Y. Li, Prospects of ceramic nanoparticles as additives for carbon-bonded MgO–C refractories, *International Journal of Applied Ceramic Technology*, 4(6), 481–489, 2007.
7. C. G. Aneziris, D. Borzov, and J. Ulbricht, Magnesia-carbon bricks: A high-duty refractory material, *Interceram—Refractories Manual*, pp. 22–27, 2003.
8. B. Brenzy, The microstructures and properties of magnesia-carbon refractories, *Key Engineering Materials*, 88, 21–40, 1993.
9. M. Guo, Degradation mechanisms of magnesia–carbon refractories by high-alumina stainless steel slags under vacuum, *Ceramics International*, 33(6), 1007–1018, 2007.
10. A. S. Gokce, C. Gurcan, S. Ozgen, and S. Aydin, The effect of antioxidants on the oxidation behaviour of magnesia–carbon refractory bricks, *Ceramics International*, 34(2), 323–330, 2008.
11. N. K. Ghosh, D. N. Ghosh, and K.P. Jagannathan, Oxidation mechanism of MgO–C in the air at various temperatures, *British Ceramic Transactions*, 99(3), 124–128, 2000.
12. S. K. Sadrnezhaad, S. Mahshid, B. Hashemi, and Z. A. Nemati, Oxidation mechanism of C in MgO–C refractory bricks, *Journal of the American Ceramic Society*, 89(4), 1308–1316, 2006.
13. N. K. Ghosh, K. P. Jagannathan, and D. N. Ghosh, Oxidation of magnesia-carbon refractories with the addition of aluminium and silicon in air, *Interceram*, 50(3), 196–202, 2001.
14. S. K. Sadrnezhaad, Z. A. Nemati, S. Mahshid, S. Hosseini, and B. Hashemi, Effect of Al antioxidant on the rate of oxidation of carbon in MgO–C refractory, *Journal of the American Ceramic Society*, 90(2), 509–515, 2007.
15. http://www.magnesita.com/refractories/steel/steelmaking/primary-refining/converters/?lang=en

CHAPTER 12

Special Refractories

THERE ARE MANY REFRACTORY items that are used industrially but with a much reduced volume. But they are also equally important as they possess some special characteristics and essentially important for certain specific applications and conditions. These materials can be termed in general as special refractories, and some of these special refractories are described here.

12.1 ZIRCON AND ZIRCONIA REFRACTORIES

Zircon ($ZrSiO_4$) is the silicate of zirconium, containing 67% ZrO_2 and 33% SiO_2. It is used as a refractory material directly and also used as a raw material for zirconia (ZrO_2). The main reason for these materials to become a refractory is the presence of zirconia in them, which is high melting, chemically inert, and imparts special mechanical properties in the refractories.

Due to its refractory character, zircon is being used and studied since long though its thermal stability, decomposition, and melting character varies from sources of origin and scientific reports. Zircons always contains some amount of hafnium; the HfO_2–ZrO_2 ratio varies but is normally about 0.01–0.04. The presence of other impurities like iron and rare earth elements are also common and also affect the decomposition and softening behavior of zircon.

Zircon has a wide range of applications as a ceramic and refractory material, for example,

- As refractory, it is mainly used for the construction of glass tank furnaces and nozzles for iron and steel industries.

- As molds and cores in precision, investment casting.

- As protective coatings on steel molding tools.

- As an opacifier in the glaze for ceramic and whiteware industries due to its high refractive index.

- As the principal precursor for the preparation of metallic zirconium and its compounds, like zirconia.

The wide range of applications of zircon is due to its excellent thermophysical properties such as low thermal expansion, good thermal stability, and high corrosion resistance against glass melts, slag, and liquid metals and alloys. Zircon is one of the most chemically stable compounds, and mineral acids other than HF cannot attack zircon. Very aggressive reaction conditions are required to break down the strong bonding between the zirconium and silicon parts of the compound.

Zircon decomposes by a solid-state reaction, and chemically pure zircon decomposes in solid state at $1676 \pm 7°C$ to form a mixture of tetragonal zirconia and cristobalite. But the presence of impurities reduces the decomposition temperature, which may even start at $1285°C$. Specifically, the more the impurities present in zircon, the lower the onset temperature of dissociation. To reduce the degree of zircon degradation, impurities, like iron, titanium, aluminum, and alkali must be minimum. Also, it is critical for the prediction of expected lifetime of zircon refractories in contact with silica-containing melts having different cations.

Zircon-based refractories are prepared by using beneficiated zircon aggregate or sand, fine-milled zircon, and a temporary binder. It is then pressed into desired shape and size, and finally the shapes are fired. The firing temperature must be lower than the decomposition temperature of zircon. The shaping of critical shapes is done by ramming, vibrocasting, or a series of air hammering technique called impact pressing. The main feature of the zircon refractories is their acidic slag resistance, excellent thermal shock resistance, and good mechanical strength with wear and erosion resistances.

Zircon refractories are used as ladle nozzles for steel pouring, tundish metering nozzles, in furnaces for melting aluminum, as compounds and coatings. Zircon refractories with at least 63% zirconia and maximum 20% apparent porosity are used in glass tank furnace. It is also an ideal mold and chill sand due to its low thermal expansion rate, high thermal conductivity, and non-wettability with molten metal. Zircon is also used in core and mould washes to improve surface finish.

Zirconia is mainly obtained by chemical processing of zircon or by carbothermal reduction (fusion) of zircon in an electric arc furnace. Also, zirconia has a natural source, called baddeleyite, commonly found in igneous rocks containing felspar, zircon, etc. Baddeleyite is chemically homogeneous, but it may contain impurities such as hafnium (Hf), titanium (Ti), and iron (Fe). Zirconia is an important refractory material due to its excellent high-temperature properties and chemical inertness. But high cost and cracking tendency have restricted its wide application.

At ambient condition, zirconia has a monoclinic structure, which instantaneously changes to tetragonal form during heating around 1180°C and from the tetragonal to the cubic form around 2370°C. On further heating, it melts around 2715°C. During cooling also, the cubic form converts to the tetragonal form at 2370°C but tetragonal changes to monoclinic at 980°C with a huge volume expansion during cooling. This spontaneous expansion during cooling (generally cooling means contraction in dimension) causes cracking and failure of the material. Hence for any high-temperature application, zirconia has to be stabilized, where additions of CaO/MgO/CeO$_2$/Y$_2$O$_3$, etc. are done to stabilize the tetragonal phase (called partially stabilized) or cubic phase (called fully stabilized) zirconia. The control on these polymorphic changes (and associated cracking) helps to incorporate microcracks within the zirconia-containing body and results in extremely high tough ceramics, which is highly beneficial for structural applications.

Zirconia refractories have refractoriness above 2000°C and also have excellent chemical resistance to the action of melts, alkalis, and most of the acids. But due to the high cost, they are only used for very specific critical applications. The main application areas are the metering nozzle in tundish (for continuous casting of steel) and inserts in the bore area in the slide gate plates (in steel ladles). In combination with carbon, it is used as a band in the subentry nozzle (SEN) to resist the corrosive attack of mold powders during continuous casting, etc. Photographs of these applications are shown in Figure 12.1. Zirconia is mostly used as a component in a refractory composition mainly to improve mechanical, corrosion, and thermal shock properties. It is also used as crucibles for melting platinum, palladium, and other metals and quartz glass, and also in the construction of nuclear reactors. Lightweight zirconia products, fibers, and granular powders are suitable for high-temperature thermal insulation. Zirconia

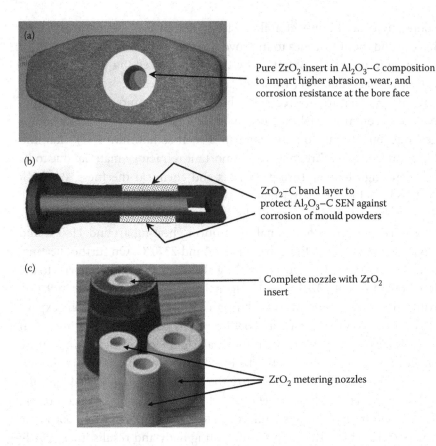

(a) Pure ZrO_2 insert in Al_2O_3–C composition to impart higher abrasion, wear, and corrosion resistance at the bore face

(b) ZrO_2–C band layer to protect Al_2O_3–C SEN against corrosion of mould powders

(c) Complete nozzle with ZrO_2 insert

ZrO_2 metering nozzles

FIGURE 12.1 Applications of zirconia in refractory: (a) as insert in slide gate plate refractory, (b) as ZrO_2–C mix in slag band of subentry nozzles, and (c) as nozzle insert in tundish nozzle.

is also used as heating elements at temperatures up to 2200°C in furnaces with resistive and induction heating.

12.2 FUSED CAST REFRACTORIES

Fused cast refractories are a different class of refractories produced by melting the raw material of the desired composition and then casting the molten mass in molds and solidified by cooling. They are widely different from conventional crystalline refractories of the similar composition due to superior corrosion resistance and the process of manufacturing.

The raw materials, generally pure oxides, are charged and melt, usually in electric arc furnaces, at temperatures above 2000°C. Sometimes induction, oxygen-gas, or plasma furnaces are also used for melting. The melt is cast in sand, graphite, or cast-iron molds of desired shapes and dimensions. The main disadvantages of graphite and metal molds are their high thermal conductivity, which may result in faster cooling at surfaces, causing stress and stress cracking at the refractory surfaces. Also, they may discolor the cast shapes surfaces. After casting, the shapes are also treated with oxygen while in the fused state to convert the constituent ions to their most highly oxidized state. Then the cast shapes are cooled slowly to solidify, even sometimes under thermal insulation. Slow cooling results in the desired large crystal sizes. In many cases, depending on the shape and size of the cast, cooling may be done for about 3–4 weeks. During cooling, a contraction cavity may be formed beneath the casting scar on the top surface of the shape and sawed to remove from the shape after cooling. The surface opposite to the casting scar is generally used as the working face. A finished work of drilling or cutting is done on the cooled shapes by grinding with diamond tools to accurately match the desired dimensions.

Fused cast refractories have a dense crystalline structure that provides superb strength, corrosion, and erosion resistances even at very high temperatures. They are quite stable against aggressive melts such as glass and molten metal oxides. Fused cast refractories have a very little amount of porosity, mostly closed pore in nature. The ingress of aggressive media cannot occur because of the low porosity and the corrosion resistant compositions. As a consequence, adhesion of slag can be prevented. Again relatively high thermal conductivity (due to dense structure) results in a uniform heat distribution within the shapes and provides better thermal shock resistances. But the thermal stability of these refractories is usually not very high. Fused cast refractories have a surface porosity of 1%–3%, compression strength in the range of 400–700 MPa and have high creep resistance.

Most of the fused cast refractories are based on the Al_2O_3–SiO_2–ZrO_2 system. The addition of other oxides like calcia, chromia, and magnesia are also done in certain cases, especially to impart any specific property or to control the crystalline structure. Based on the mineralogical composition, fused cast refractories are classified as follows.

12.2.1 Fused Cast Alumina Refractories

Fuse cast alumina refractories contain more than 90% Al_2O_3 and have excellent resistance to acidic slag and chemical corrosion. According to the crystallographic analysis, fused cast alumina refractories are commonly classified as alpha-fused cast alumina, beta-fused cast alumina,

TABLE 12.1   Classification of Fused Cast Alumina Refractories

Types	Soda Content (wt%)	Beta Alumina Content (vol%)
Fused α-alumina	<1.1	<10
Fused α-β alumina	3.5–4.7	50–65
Fused β-alumina	5.2–7.7	>95
Fused β″-alumina	4.5 (~8 MgO)	>95 as β″ ($NaMg_2Al_{15}O_{25}$)

and alpha–beta fused cast alumina. As per ASTM C 1547-02 (2013), these refractories are classified as per their soda (Na_2O) content, as obtained from chemical analysis and the beta (β) alumina ($NaAl_{11}O_{17}$) or beta″ (β″) alumina ($NaMg_2Al_{15}O_{25}$) phases content, as obtained from quantitative phase analysis (by x-ray diffraction) or image analysis study. Table 12.1 shows the details of the classification. Neutral character of fused cast alumina against alkali vapors makes it the best choice for the downstream part of superstructures in glass tank furnaces.

12.2.2 Fused Cast Al_2O_3–ZrO_2–SiO_2 (AZS) Refractories

Fused cast Al_2O_3–ZrO_2–SiO_2 refractories, abbreviated as AZS, are important for their corrosion resistance and wear properties mainly due to its compositions and considerable ZrO_2 content in them. They are the most widely used materials both in glass contact areas and superstructure of glass melting furnaces due to their very high resistances against glass and alkali vapor.

These refractories are further divided as per ZrO_2 content. According to ASTM C 1547-02 (2013), these refractories are classified by the amount of monoclinic zirconia (ZrO_2) present, as determined by chemical analysis or quantitative image analysis. Table 12.2 shows the details of the classifications.

12.2.3 Fused Cast Zirconia Refractories

The fused cast zirconia refractories contain at least 80% of ZrO_2 and have excellent corrosion and wear resistance against molten glass. Therefore,

TABLE 12.2   Classification of Fused Cast Alumina–Zirconia–Silica (AZS) and Fused Cast Zirconia Refractories

Types	Zirconia Content (wt%)	Zirconia Content (vol%)
AZS 21	19–23	18.5–22.5
AZS 33	31–34	30.5–33.5
AZS 36	34.5–37.5	34–37
AZS 40	38–41	37.5–41
Zirconia	>90	>90

it has been widely used in contact with molten glass in a glass melting furnaces.

12.2.4 Fused Cast Alumina–Zirconia Refractories

Fused cast alumina–zirconia refractories are important for their high strength, excellent resistances against wear and slag corrosion as well as long service life. They are mainly used in areas that require high abrasion and temperature resistance, such as gliding rail bricks in steel pusher metallurgical furnaces, the tapping platform style walking beam furnaces, etc.

12.2.5 Fused Cast Alumina–Silica Refractories

Fused cast alumina–silica refractories are characterized by excellent resistance to high temperatures, acid corrosion, erosion, and thermal shocks. They show high performance on reheating furnace beds, skid rails, and for the linings of industrial waste incinerators. It is widely used in the metallurgical and glass industries, ceramic kilns, and the cement industry. ASTM C 1547-02 (2013) classifies (shown in Table 12.3) these refractories as per their alumina content and alumina to silica (Al_2O_3:SiO_2) ratio, as determined by chemical analysis using quantitative phase analysis or image analysis study.

Fused cast refractories are the preferred refractories in contact with glass melts, due to their chemical stability, impermeability, and resistance to corrosion and erosion at the working temperatures of the glass melting furnaces. These refractories are used in glass melting and heating furnaces, petrochemical industries, and the most vulnerable sections of metallurgical industries, like oxygen–Bessemer converter linings. Powdered fused refractories are used to make critical parts and as fillers in linings of many furnaces, including induction furnaces.

12.3 INSULATING REFRACTORIES

Insulating refractories are thermal barriers for any high-temperature processing that do not allow the heat to escape from the desired processing and save energy. Any high-temperature processing demands maximum heat conservation so as to minimize heat losses for maximum utilization

TABLE 12.3 Classification of Fused Cast Alumina–Silica Refractories

Types	Alumina Content (wt%)	Alumina:Silica Ratio
Mullite–corundum	>67	>3.6
Mullite–corundum–ZrO_2	>67 (>3 zirconia)	>3.6

of the heat charged. This will result in minimum fuel consumption as well as high production as a result of maintaining high working temperatures. As the cost of energy has increased, the role of insulating refractories has become more important.

The function of insulating refractory is to restrict or at least reduce the rate of heat flow out from the high-temperature process to the open environment. Although it is not possible to completely prevent the loss of heat when a temperature gradient exists between two surfaces but the use of insulating refractory can greatly reduce the loss and make the process energy efficient.

Heat can be transferred from one place to another by three different mechanisms, namely conduction, convection, and radiation. For solid materials, conductivity is the main mode of heat transfer. In conduction mode, heat is transferred by the transfer of energy from one atom to another (or molecule to molecule) in a material where atoms at higher temperature vibrate faster due to higher energy level and pass on the energy to the adjacent atoms present in a lower energy state (lower temperature).

So it is very common to design for an insulating refractory using a material that has a lower thermal conductivity. But in actual case, the common refractories have thermal conductivity values in a very narrow range, varies between 1 and 3 W/m K. So only by changing the refractory material, the effect on insulation will be marginal. To improve the thermal insulation character of refractories, air is incorporated as pores within the refractory body, as air has a very low thermal conductivity (~0.02 W/m K). So a refractory having high porosity will have significantly low conductivity values due to the presence of air within it. Generally, the dense commercial refractories have surface porosity of 18%–24% and total porosity in the range of 30%–35%. Incorporation of air by creating porosity in insulating refractory increases this total porosity level to the tune of 80%. But this increased insulation property is at the cost of lowering of strength, and resistances against corrosion, abrasion, etc. properties. As the insulating refractories have deteriorated mechanical, thermomechanical, and corrosion properties, they are not used in the hot face or contact with the high-temperature processing environment. Rather they are used as a backup, behind the strong and dense refractory, only to retain the heat within the system and reduce the heat loss. So, as the highest temperature that an insulating refractory encounters is the cooler side (lowest) temperature of the hot face refractory, the temperature is much lower than the actual high-temperature processing. So the refractoriness and other thermomechanical properties required are not that stringent to that of the hot face refractories. Hence generally cheap and commonly available fire clay-based insulating refractories are mostly used unless otherwise specified or required for any specific property requirement.

The structure of insulating refractory has minute pores filled up with air. The air inside the brick prevents the heat from being conducted, but the solid particles conduct the heat. So, to have the required insulation property in a brick along with other structural properties, a balance has to be made between the proportion of its solid particles and air spaces. Again higher the porosity, greater will be the insulating effect, but the size of the pore must be fine and they must be uniformly distributed. As a bigger-sized pore will have a greater volume of air, which again transfers the heat by convection mechanism within itself from the hotter side to the cooler side and heat transfer will occur. Again non-uniform distribution of porosity may result in the conduction of heat through the solid particles where porosity is less. Hence, evenly distributed small-sized pores are desirable for the best insulating character.

Generally, the porosity within the refractory is intentionally created by the addition of fine organic materials to the mix, such as sawdust, straw, rice husk, etc. during mixing process of manufacturing. Then the mix is pressed, dried carefully, and fired. Organic materials are combustible in nature and burn out during firing of the refractories, creating internal pores. There are some special ways also to create porosity within the refractory, generally used to get a high level of porosity for special purposes only. These are

1. Use of special materials that expand and open up on firing

2. Use of volatile organic materials like naphthalene, polystyrene, starch, etc.

3. Use of chemical bloating technique (like the combination of aluminum powder with NaOH solution)

4. Use of porous or open textured materials like vermiculite, ex-foliated mica, diatomite, insulating grog, etc.

5. Use of foaming agents, etc.

Insulating refractories can be classified by many aspects, like raw materials used, major oxide (constituent) present and its content, porosity, and strength level. But the common and widely acceptable method of classification is based on their heat withstanding capacity, described as follows.

1. Insulating refractories that can withstand temperature up to 1000°C. In this category, calcium silicate, siliceous earth materials, perlite or vermiculite, etc. are important.

2. Insulating refractories up to an application temperature of 1400°C. The common examples are lightweight fire clays, alumino silicates, lightweight castables, ceramic fibers, etc.

3. High-temperature insulating refractory that can withstand up to 1600°C. The examples are lightweight mullite and alumina, hollow sphere corundum (bubble alumina), alumina fibers, etc.

4. Ultrahigh-temperature insulating refractory that can withstand up to 1800°C. Porous zirconia, non-oxide compounds, etc. are common examples.

The main advantages of insulating refractories are the following:

1. They reduce the heat losses through the furnace lining and make the high-temperature processes energy efficient.

2. They allow rapid heat-up and cooling of the furnace and lowers heat capacity of the lining.

3. Thinner refractory lining can be designed with desirable thermal profile.

4. Reduction in furnace weight and thermal mass due to lower density.

But there are many disadvantages also, given as follows.

1. Insulating refractories are poor in strength due to high porosity, causing a problem in structural design.

2. They are very weak in chemical resistance due to the porous structure, causing penetration of gasses, fumes, liquids such as slags, and molten glass at high temperatures.

3. These refractories are weak against thermal spalling as higher thermal gradient exists between the hot and cold surfaces (due to lower conductivity) and lower strength values.

The applications of insulating refractories range from laboratory furnaces to foundry furnaces and large tunnel kilns. Insulating refractories are very common as backup lining in most of the high-temperature operations where strength, abrasion, and wear by aggressive slag and molten metal are not at all a concern. These are widely used in the crowns of glass furnace, and tunnel kiln applications.

12.4 CERAMIC FIBERS

Ceramic fibers are also a class of insulating materials that can be spun and fabricated into textiles, blankets, felts, boards, blocks, or any other desired shapes. Ceramic fibers have low thermal conductivity and heat storage, light weight, relatively resistant to thermal shocks, and are chemically stable. The fluffy nature of the material prevents heat loss to a great extent and allows a very high rate of heating and cooling of the furnace and kiln with high energy efficiency.

The main advantages of the ceramic fibers are as follows:

1. Better fuel economy due to low thermal mass, reduced heat storage and better heat insulation

2. Higher productivity for the user industry due to faster heating and cooling sequences

3. Longer lining life with reduced maintenance costs

4. Ease of installation

The main disadvantages of these materials are as follows:

1. Shrinkage at high temperatures and even on prolonging heating, causing open up (gap) of the refractory lining

2. Poor mechanical strength (requires proper support for any design and structural use)

3. Sagging at high temperature due to softening tendency if proper support is not provided

4. Cannot withstand any presence of liquids like slag, glass, and molten metals

5. Expensive than conventional refractories

The most common ceramic fiber systems are Al_2O_3, Al_2O_3–SiO_2, and ZrO_2. Conventionally, ceramic fibers are made by blending the purer variety of raw materials followed by melting. Melting temperature may vary between 1800°C and 2400°C depending upon the composition. Molten stream is then broken by blowing compressed air or dropping the melt on the spinning disk to form loose or bulk ceramic fiber. The bulk fiber is then converted to various shapes like blanket, strips, veneering and anchored modules, paper, vacuum formed boards and shapes, rope, wet felt, and mastic cement for various insulation applications. Different shapes made up of ceramic fibers, conventionally used for refractories, are shown in Figure 12.2.

Fibers with less than 60% Al_2O_3 are made from alumina, quartz, and zircon and are directly extracted from the electrically fused melts. The melt stream is converted to the fiber by using oppositely moving quick rotating disks or by high-speed air jet blowing sideways (parallel) to the molten stream. These fibers have a glassy structure due to faster cooling. Again fibers with more than 60% alumina, difficult to produce by conventional melting route, are extracted from spinning solutions containing aluminum and silicon with some organic carrier (melting process requires

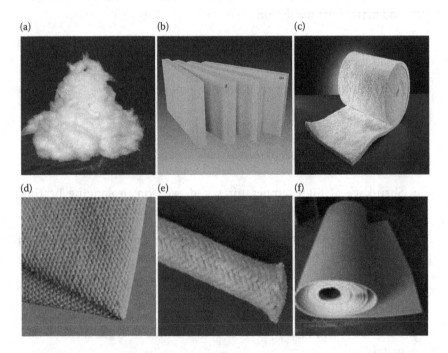

FIGURE 12.2 Different forms and shapes of ceramic fibers generally used in refractories: (a) bulk fiber, (b) board, (c) blanket, (d) cloth, (e) rope, and (f) paper.

much higher temperature and energy for processing). The spinner materials are then heat-treated to remove the organic material first and then further heat-treated to convert the fibers into solid stable state.

Due to prolonged service or excessive temperatures, the structure of the fibers change and the glassy fibers convert to mullite and cristobalite. This is associated with changes in volume and strength. Originally the smooth surfaced fiber becomes rough; the crystal appears, and the fibers become brittle. From the shrinkage parameter of the fibers, due to the structural change, the fibers are classified according to the maximum permissible application temperature. The maximum temperature that a fiber can withstand without shrinking 4% linearly when heated from all the sides for 24 h is called the classification temperature. Obviously, a higher alumina-containing fiber has a higher classification temperature and can be applied at higher temperatures.

Ceramic fibers are widely used for metal treatment furnaces, ceramic kilns, and many periodic heating operations. Fibers are common in expansion joints, door seals, preventing any heat leakage in any high-temperature applications. These materials can be directly used as hot face refractory where liquid corrosion or penetration and strength requirements are not the major requirements. Shapes made from fibers containing 52% Al_2O_3 and 48% SiO_2 are important for hot face insulation up to 1400°C. Higher the alumina content, higher is the application temperature. Pure Al_2O_3 and ZrO_2 fibers and their shapes are used even up to 1800°C.

12.5 CARBON REFRACTORIES

Carbon refractories behave differently than the typical oxide refractories, as carbon is a conductive material rather than insulating. They essentially consist of elemental carbon as the major constituent. The application areas of these refractories must be such that the presence of oxygen or air will be minimum. Otherwise the carbon will oxidize and burn out. Many a time, carbon and graphite are used to represent the same material, but precisely carbon is a general term that represents many carbon-bearing sources in which graphite is also one natural source.

The main advantages of carbon as refractory are as follows:

1. High refractory character with thermal stability in non-oxidizing conditions

2. Poor wettability by polar liquids, in particular by silicate-based slags

3. Potentially high thermal conductivity

4. Low thermal expansion properties

5. Excellent thermal shock resistance characteristics

In nature, carbon is available in several forms, the most common ones being diamond, graphite, and amorphous carbon. Diamond is a precious stone and insulating in character. Graphite is a crystalline, black, hexagonal layer network structured very soft material, conducts heat and electricity, and shows lubricity. Amorphous carbon has hexagonal layers like graphite but with disordered stacking and results in amorphous character; but it is a hard material. Coke and charcoal do not have distinct crystalline character and have properties in between a graphite and a diamond. Varieties of properties coming from the same carbon material are due to the variation of carbon atom arrangements and its nature of bonding.

The raw materials used for making carbon refractories are petroleum coke, natural and synthetic graphite (both the crystalline and amorphous forms), pitch coke, metallurgical coke, and calcined anthracite. These materials act as fillers for the carbon refractory and pitch, tar, and resin are used as binders. Metal additives are also used as antioxidants and also some other additives are added to enhance certain properties.

Among different sources, graphite is preferred by the refractory industries mainly due to its greater oxidation resistance, coming from its low porosity level. Oxidation can only occur through the active sites in the granular planes. Also, flakiness (aspect ratio) is high for graphite, and so flaky graphite is preferred for its high thermal conductivity. Thus helps in further higher thermal shock resistances. But higher flakiness enhances the chances of lamination and anisotropic character. There is also an amorphous variety of graphite, which is found in nature in a massive form. But natural graphite contains ash (about 8%–15%), which drastically degrades the properties. The ash contains about 45%–50% silica, 15%–20% alumina, 15%–25% iron oxides, little alkalis, and alkaline earth oxides. Natural graphite is required to be cleaned, washed, and purified (using floatation process) to reduce the impurities content (resulting in ash) before use. Synthetic graphite is also used for making carbon refractories, generally produced from the used graphite electrodes, which are crushed to get the desired fractions. Synthetic graphite is purer and has higher thermal conductivity but dissolves easily in molten iron.

Petroleum coke is the calcined form of the green coke obtained from the petroleum industries. Crude petroleum is decomposed and distilled to separate out the precious gasses, oils, and other petroleum products and the remaining residue is the green coke. This green coke is calcined about 1200°C to produce the petroleum coke. Also, the pitch coke is obtained in the same manner. The main advantage of these cokes is that they have very low ash content. Metallurgical coke of foundry variety is preferred for refractories due to its higher mechanical properties and abrasion resistances.

Anthracite is also used as a major ingredient for carbon refractories after calcination in reducing conditions. Natural anthracite contains a good amount of volatile matter and ash content. Calcination can be accompolished by gas firing or electrical firing. Gas-fired calcination process is done around 1200°C, and the calcined anthracite has better mechanical properties but poor thermal and shrinkage characteristics. Electrical calcination is done in a wide range of temperatures, varying from 1200°C to 2500°C. The calcination temperature affects the properties of the product, likes volume stability, electrical and thermal conductivity, strength, abrasion, and alkali resistances.

Raw materials as per desired size fractions are mixed with hot tar or pitch, and the mixing temperature is maintained about 50°C higher than the softening temperature of the binder, for better flowability and mixing. Any lump formation is avoided for a uniform texture of the mix. Mixed paste is then shaped by extrusion or by pouring into molds and then further shaping. Extrusion is done at around 100–120°C and used mainly for the bulk production of dense shapes (low porosity) even at a lower binder content. There are chances of aggregate alignment in the extrusion direction and anisotropic character in the shaped products. Molding is done around 70–100°C and gives a relatively isotropic character in the shapes. Shapes can be rammed for better compaction in the hot condition and finally allowed to cool. Green shapes are then fired (baked) in the absence of air. They are first packed in coke to avoid oxidation and deformation due to softening on heating. This baking is done around 1300°C with a slow heating and cooling schedule, heating for 2–3 weeks, and cooling for about a week. For graphite-containing compositions, the temperature used is much higher than the simple baking temperature. For compositions containing synthetic graphite, the firing temperature is further higher, and a graphitization process (at 2500°C) is followed by baking to increase the strength and thermal conductivity of the products. Baked or graphitized refractories are finally cut and machined to match the required dimensions.

The properties of carbon refractories vary widely depending upon the raw materials used for making them. Bulk density varies between 1.5 and

1.8 g/cm^3 and apparent porosity is in the range of 12%–25%. They all have poor oxidation resistance but very high thermal stability if oxidation is controlled. The cold strength varies between 40 and 100 MPa, and linear reheat change is negative within 1% at 1500°C (higher values for metallurgical coke). RUL values under 0.2 MPa load is above 1750°C if oxidation can be restricted. Abrasion resistance is again dependent on the raw materials used. Graphite-containing compositions have higher thermal conductivity but are softer and results in high abrasion loss compared to coke-based products. Carbon refractory based on electrographite has about 25 times higher conductivity than metallurgical coke-based ones at 200°C and about 10 times higher at 800°C. The bonding characteristics and flakiness of graphite have resulted in such a high thermal conductivity value. Carbon refractories are weak against oxidation, which is caused by oxygen and carbon dioxide present in the environment and also by the moisture present (leaking coolers). Carbon refractories are hardly attacked by molten slag and metal as they have a non-wetting character due to strong covalent bonding among the atoms. The presence of alkalis is detrimental to carbon as they may react and form intercalation compounds (say C16K, C24K, etc.). These compound formations are associated with growth, expansion, and result in disintegration of the refractory.

The blast furnace is the largest user of carbon refractories followed by aluminum industries. Anthracite- and graphite-based carbon refractories are mainly useful for the hearth and bosh portion of the blast furnace. Carbon refractories are also important for the lower stack runners of a blast furnace. For blast furnace, bosh area and high thermal conductivity with abrasion resistance is required. Metallurgical coke-based products show good abrasion resistance, but they have low thermal conductivity, whereas electrographite-based refractories have a very high thermal conductivity but poor abrasion resistance. For blast furnace applications, high resistance against abrasion is essential, so softer refractories are not preferred. However, the formation of slag coating on the refractory surface reduces the abrasion effect on the refractory and softer ones also perform well. This slag coating forms easily for refractories with high thermal conductivity. In aluminum industries, petroleum coke and amorphous carbon–based refractories are useful as anodes, cathodes, sidewalls, and hearth of the smelters. Graphite refractories are also important for various ferroalloys industries like Fe–Si, Fe–Cr and Fe–Mo. Graphite–alumina and graphite–aluminosilicate refractories are important for various areas of steel and non-ferrous metal industries.

12.6 SILICON CARBIDE REFRACTORIES

Silicon carbide (SiC) refractories are important as they exhibit a unique combination of properties, like high strength both at ambient and elevated temperatures, high thermal conductivity, and high resistances against thermal shock, abrasion, erosion, and corrosion of non-oxidizing slags and metals. SiC is prepared by the well-known Acheson process (about 125 years old) where quartz and coke are intimately mixed and heated for days in a special electric resistance furnace. Carbothermal reduction of silica ($SiO_2 + 3C = SiC + 2CO$) occurs at about 1600–2300°C. The process of making SiC and the furnace design have remained nearly unchanged since its inception in 1893. In a typical commercial process, about 150 ton of batch material is used (mix of quartz and coke) and about 150 MWh of electrical energy is required to produce about 15 tons of SiC and the remaining batch materials were again reused in subsequent processes. SiC chunks obtained from the process are crushed and graded as per the desired fractions for different uses.

Silicon carbide is a light weight, a very hard abrasion resistant material with a thermal conductivity of 21 W/m K at 1000°C. It is resistant to dilute acids and alkalis but decomposes in fused alkali carbonates, borax, and cryolite. Also, SiC dissociates into Si and C in molten iron and steel and oxidizes in the air above 800°C but stable up to 2200°C in reducing atmosphere. The use of SiC initially began as an abrasive material due to its excellent hardness and as on today, it is the second largest used abrasive material. Grains and powders are important as polishing, lapping, and shot-blasting material and also used for grinding wheels, finishing stones, coated abrasives like fiber disk, etc. They are also used as metallurgical additives as inoculants for cast iron and deoxidizer for steel. Sintered shapes are also used as electrical heating elements, mechanical seal, lightning arrestor, and igniter.

The use of silicon carbide in refractories has started about the 1970s since its use in a blast furnace. SiC is a strong covalently bonded solid and as a refractory the main advantages of SiC are as follows:

- Light weight (bulk density <3 g/cm³)
- High strength at high temperatures (up to 1600°C)
- Excellent thermal stability and thermal shock resistance
- High thermal conductivity and low electrical conductivity

- Resistance to oxidation (among non-oxides), corrosion, abrasion, and erosion

- Resistance to molten non-ferrous metals and slags

As SiC is a very strongly bonded material (about 89% covalent bonding), it has weak diffusivity and difficult to get sintered. Hence, for making any shaped product of SiC very high temperature and pressure are required or a secondary material is to be added as a sintering aid. Again at high temperatures, the surface of SiC is covered with an incipient layer of silica (due to oxidation), different bond formations can be designed, for getting better sintered products, by the addition of proper additive utilizing this silica layer. But the final properties of the sintered SiC products are dependent on the bond types and are detailed in Table 12.4. Different types of bond used in SiC refractories are as follows.

- Oxide bonded [OB-SiC]

- Nitride bonded [NB-SiC]

- Reaction {self-bonded} [RB-SiC]

- Direct sintered [DS-SiC]

Oxide-bonded (OB) SiC are based on silica or silicate phases formed during firing due to oxidative or glass forming reactions. Addition of clay, silica, and mullite is done with SiC batch composition, and the mixture is shaped by pressing, vibrocasting, and pneumatic ramming and then fired

TABLE 12.4　Variations in Properties of SiC Refractories with Different Bonding Systems

Sl.	Property	OB-SiC	NB-SiC	RB-SiC	DS-SiC
1	Bulk density (g/cm³)	2.3–2.5	2.5–2.7	2.7–3.1	3.0–3.1
2	App. porosity (%)	15–25	15–18	<1	1–3
3	HOT MoR at 1250°C (MPa)	18–25	45–80	300–450	550–650
4	Thermal expansion coefficient $\times 10^{-6}/°C$	5.3–5.9	4.0–5.0	4.3–4.6	4.0–4.2
5	Thermal conductivity (W/m K)	8–12	15–30	90–115	90–100
6	Thermal shock resistance	Good	V. good	Excellent	Excellent
7	Oxidation resistance	Fair	V. good	V. good	Excellent
8	Corrosion resistance	Fair	V. good	V. good	Excellent
9	Abrasion resistance	Good	Excellent	V. good	V. good

in an oxidizing atmosphere. Oxide ingredients react with the incipient silica layer formed on SiC surface and develops the bond. The amount and nature of bond and the developed properties can be tailored by the amount and type of the additions done. Generally, the hot strength is strongly affected due to the presence of the liquid phase at high temperatures. Amount of SiC present in the final refractories is around 80%.

Nitride-bonded silicon carbide refractories is a general name given to products containing nitride bond [NB-SiC], oxy-nitride bond [ONB-SiC], and SiAlON bond [SAB-SiC]. As per the desired bond in the final ceramics silicon metal powder; silicon metal powder and fume silica; and silicon metal powder and fine alumina powders are added respectively to different fractions of SiC batch materials. Conventional shaping techniques are used, and firing is done in a nitrogen atmosphere at around 1550°C (close to melting point of metallic silicon). During firing, the nitrogen gas reacts with silicon metal forming silicon nitride (Si_3N_4), and these nitrides get accommodated in the porous structure of the shape. Hence for silicon metal–containing composition, the dimensional change is very marginal. However, there is a significant increase in the weight. The NB–SiC product has a fibrous matrix of silicon nitride (and small amounts of oxy-nitride) in which SiC grains are strongly held. In oxy-nitride bonded material, formed silicon nitride further reacts with silica and form SiON phase in the fired shapes. Whereas the compositions containing both silicon powder and alumina, the formed Si_3N_4 reacts with alumina, forming SiAlON. In ONB and SAB-SiC bonded products, a thin film of SiO_2 is always present on the surface of SiC grains. NB–SiC refractories have a minimum SiC content of 75%.

In reaction-bonded (RB) SiC refractories, different fractions of SiC are mixed with fine graphite, pressed and fired in a vacuum capable or environment controlled furnace between 1500 and 1650°C. Granular silicon metal is placed in contact with the shapes at the high temperatures that melts and wets the SiC shapes and wicks through the compacts. During this process, an exothermic reaction occurs due to the reaction between silicon melt and graphite forming nascent secondary SiC phase that acts as a bond material in the shape. Firing conditions along with amount of free graphite and silicon metal melt to be provided are required to be precisely controlled to control the formation of reaction bonding within the shape. These refractories contain at least 90% SiC in its composition.

Direct sintered (DS) or self-bonded SiC refractories are prepared from a mixture of submicron-sized SiC powders with sintering aids like boron and aluminum. Organic binders and resin, as a source of carbon, are also used in the composition. The compositions are shaped by casting or pressing and fired in a controlled atmosphere vacuum furnace at 2000–2200°C. These refractories have very high shrinkage (20%), due to high sintering, good density, and excellent high strength properties and contain about 99% SiC in its composition.

Applications of SiC refractories are mainly in the blast furnace linings, especially in the tuyere band, bosh, belly, and lower and middle stack. The upper stack region has a low temperature but is under high wear due to abrasion of the solid batch materials, and OB-SiC refractories are used. In lower stack and belly portion, along with abrasion and alkali vapor attack, higher temperatures are also important, and NB-SiC refractories are preferred. Further increase in temperature with greater alkali and zinc attack and corrosion from molten metal and slag are important in the bosh region, and SiAlON-bonded SiC refractories are suitable for such critical environments.

NB–SiC refractories are also used for the lining of Hall cells in primary aluminum production through Hall–Heroult process where highly corrosive cryolite liquid is present. SiC refractories are also used in the secondary melting of aluminum, like walls of reverberatory remelting furnaces and immersed radiant tubes. SiC refractories, generally OB-SiC types, are also important as backup lining for the hot face carbon refractories in the tap hole region of electric arc furnaces used in ferro alloy industries. They help to control the metal viscosity due to its high thermal conductivity and act as heat sink. For the higher abrasion and corrosion resistances, NB-SiC refractories are used as lining for the reverberatory holding furnaces for copper melting. Also different shapes of OB-SiC refractories are used in a vertical fractional distillation column to purify zinc from impure natural sources.

SiC refractories are also used as kiln furniture in the insulator, sanitary ware, tiles, and table ware industries in the shapes of batts, plates, tiles, pillars, saggers, etc. SiC refractories are important due to the high-temperature stability, strength, creep resistances, high thermal conductivity, and thermal shock resistances. These refractories allow high ware (being fired) to kiln furniture weight ratio, and improves productivity and fuel efficiency. Different bonding systems are used for these applications depending on the application demand and properties achieved. Figure 12.3 shows the applications of SiC-based shapes as kiln furniture.

(a)

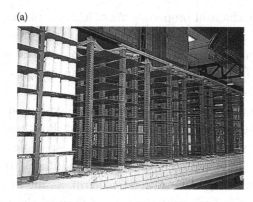

(b)

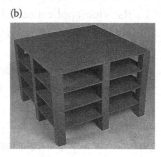

FIGURE 12.3 Use of SiC as a kiln furniture (a) on the tunnel kiln car where products are being fired and (b) an assembly of kiln furniture to make rack or shelf using SiC support rods and plates/batts.

12.7 OTHER NON-OXIDES IN REFRACTORIES

Continuous development and improvement of metallurgical industries, especially the iron and steelmaking technology, have demanded refractories to cope up with the advancements and provide the desired performances in further stringent environments, maintaining both the environmental and economic factors. Though refractory comes under the broad classification of traditional ceramics, these high-performance refractories need to have certain specific application-oriented properties that cannot be obtained from the conventional compositions. Hence, the refractory researchers are always in search of newer materials that can provide very specific properties essential for a particular application. These new materials also expected to enhance the performance and service life greatly. These special additives are mostly non-oxide in nature and are commercially used in a very small fraction (volume) to the total refractory required or used. Mostly they have excellent structural or mechanical characteristics and mainly incorporated in refractories to improve the structural properties. Few of these non-oxides are discussed in the following.

12.7.1 Boron Carbide (B_4C)

Boron carbide is the hardest material after diamond, so it shows excellent abrasion and wear resistance. It has a good corrosion resistance, especially against the acids. Generally, it is associated with some amount of free carbon, as secondary graphite phase and has a purity in the range of 78%–85%.

This free carbon affects the mechanical properties. Also, it is low in oxidation resistance compared to silicon carbide, and low fracture toughness limits its wide applications. In commercial production, boron carbide is manufactured by reacting and fusing boric oxide with carbon in an electric arc furnace.

B_4C is a strong covalent-bonded material, so to get a high dense product hot pressing (or hot isostatic pressing) technique is used. But these special manufacturing techniques restrict the dimensions and complexity of shapes and costly cutting and grinding (using diamond tools) are required. The interesting properties of B_4C are extreme hardness and low thermal conductivity, resulting in high brittleness, poor thermal shock resistances; good thermal-neutron absorbance, and high wear resistance. Some of the properties are listed in Table 12.5.

It is used extensively as ballistic armor and blast nozzles and is the primary choice for control rods and other nuclear applications, abrasive as lapping and ultrasonic cutting, armor materials, wire drawing dies, powder metal and ceramic forming dies, and thread guides. As a refractory, B_4C is important as an antioxidant in $MgO-C$ refractory as it oxidizes at much lower temperature compared to conventional metallic antioxidants and protects carbon. Also, it is important as a component in nozzles for flow control of hot aggressive liquids.

12.7.2 Tungsten Carbide (WC)

Tungsten carbide is a very hard wear resistance material mostly important for industrial machinery, cutting tools, abrasives, armors, and so on. Generally, it contains high percentages of either cobalt or nickel as a second metallic phase. These ceramic materials behave like a metal and also called "ceramic metals" or "cermets." Tungsten carbide is prepared by reaction of tungsten metal and carbon between 1400°C and 2000°C or by using a fluidized bed process that reacts either tungsten metal or blue

TABLE 12.5 Properties of Some Metal Carbides Useful for Refractory Industries

Material	Density (g/cm³)	Melting Point (°C)	Thermal Expansion Coefficient (10^{-6}°C^{-1})	Thermal Conductivity (W/m K)	Microhardness (MPa)	Elastic Modulus (GPa)
B_4C	2.52	2350	4.5	0.3	3340	1.5
WC	15.5	2720	3.8	0.07	1780	8.1
TiC	4.9	3100	7.7	25	3300	4.6
ZrC	6.9	3530	6.7	0.05	2930	3.5

WO_3 with CO/CO_2 mixture and H_2 between 900°C and 1200°C. Shapes of pure tungsten carbide can be made as an advanced technical ceramic using a high-temperature hot isostatic pressing process. This material has very high hardness and wear resistance and is mainly used as a cutting tool, grinding media, abrasive water jet nozzles; however, its weight limits the use in many applications. Some properties of sintered WC products are shown in Table 12.5.

Tungsten carbide compositions have outstanding physical and mechanical properties, good impact strength, outstanding dimensional stability, exceptional heat resistance and resistance to thermal shock, good cryogenic properties and oxidation resistances up to ~600°C, and even good tensile strength. In refractory, it is used to impart high wear and abrasion resistance for critical application areas.

12.7.3 Silicon Nitride (Si_3N_4)

Si_3N_4 has the strongest covalent bond properties next to silicon carbide. It is used as a high-temperature structural ceramic due to its superior heat resistance, strength, and hardness. It also offers excellent wear and corrosion resistance. Its high strength and toughness make it the material of choice for automotive and bearing applications.

Silicon nitride can be made by heating powdered silicon powder in a nitrogen atmosphere in the temperature range of 1300–1400°C.

$$3Si + 2N_2 \rightarrow Si_3N_4$$

Due to the attachment of nitrogen with silicon, the weight of the sample increases with time and the formation completes with a soaking time of 7 h. It is difficult to produce in bulk, and it dissociates into constituent ions on heating about 1850°C, much lower than its melting point. For shaped products of silicon nitride, bonding is done by adding sintering aids that promote liquid phase sintering and densify at lower temperatures but with a compromise of the high-temperature properties. Silicon nitride has long been used in high-temperature applications and is capable of withstanding tremendous thermal shock and thermal gradients generated in hydrogen–oxygen rocket engines. Some of the properties of sintered silicon nitride are given in Table 12.6. Various types silicon nitride–sintered shapes, produced by different methods, are useful for heat exchangers, rotors, nozzles, bearings, valves, chemical plant parts, engine components, and armor.

TABLE 12.6   Properties of Some Metal Nitrides Used in Refractory Industries

Material	Density (g/cm³)	Melting Point (°C)	Thermal Expansion Coefficient (10^{-6}°C^{-1})	Thermal Conductivity (W/m K)	Knoop Hardness (Kg mm^{-2})	Elastic Modulus (GPa)
Si_3N_4	3.18	1900	3.3	22	2200	300
AlN	3.25	2200	5	125	1170	308
BN	2.27	3000	0.7	35	150	8

12.7.4 Aluminum Nitride (AlN)

Aluminum nitride is mainly important for the semiconductor industries and relatively newer material in the technical ceramics family. In its pure form, it is white in color and any tan, or gray coloration indicates contaminations. It is a covalently bonded material with a hexagonal crystal structure and requires sintering aids even in hot pressing technique. Oxidation starts at the surface from about 700°C in the air, which forms alumina on the surface and protects the material up to about 1370°C, above which rapid oxidation occurs. But AlN is very stable in inert atmospheres. It is attacked slowly by mineral acids and strong alkalis and it also hydrolyzes slowly in water. The key features of aluminum nitride are high thermal conductivity, low thermal expansion, and also low electrical conductivity. Some of the properties of sintered AlN are given in Table 12.6. The main application areas are molten metal handling components, material processing kiln furniture, heat sinks, and substrates for electronic packages.

12.7.5 Boron Nitride (BN)

Hexagonal boron nitride is a white chalky material and is often called the "white graphite." It has poor mechanical properties. There are different varieties of boron nitrides available, and nearly all of them show outstanding high-temperature resistance (>2500°C) in inert atmospheres but oxidizes above 800°C in an air atmosphere. BN shapes are made by hot pressing technique and can be machined using standard carbide drills. Due to its crystal structure, BN is anisotropic electrically and mechanically. BN composites show excellent thermal shock resistance, corrosion resistance to molten metals and chemicals, strain and damage tolerance, wear resistance, and machinability. Some of the properties of sintered BN are shown in Table 12.6. BN is used as vacuum components, low-friction seals, various electronic parts, nuclear applications, and plasma arc insulators. It is also used as a high-temperature insulator and in combination with TiB_2 in many ferrous and aluminum metallurgical applications.

12.7.6 Metal Borides

Among different metal borides, titanium diboride (TiB_2) and zirconium diboride (ZrB_2) are important. Both the borides are prepared by the carbothermal reduction of the respective oxides in the presence of B_2O_3, which is an economic and traditional process. Above 1000°C, the B_2O_3 volatilizes and forms the borides as per the following equations.

$$ZrO_2 + B_2O_3 + C \rightarrow ZrB_2 + 5CO$$
$$TiO_2 + B_2O_3 + C \rightarrow TiB_2 + 5CO$$

The products of TiB_2 and ZrB_2 are commonly sintered by hot pressing technique under vacuum or inert atmosphere. But at ambient pressure, it takes about 1900–2200°C in a controlled atmosphere in the presence of sintering additives like metals, carbon, and rare earth oxides. Both the borides have a high melting point, low electrical resistance, high hardness, high thermal conductivity, and excellent corrosion resistance up to 1100°C. They are resistant to HCl and HF but are weak and decompose in alkali metal hydrate. Some of the properties of these borides are shown in Table 12.7.

They are widely used as hard tools and cutting tools, wire stretching mold, and sand jetting nozzle. Both of them are important as high-temperature refractories (2000–3000°C) when the atmosphere is not oxidizing in nature. Titanium diboride is used in metallurgical applications involving molten aluminum. It is also used for some limited wear applications, such as ballistic armor to stop large-diameter (>14.5 mm) projectiles. TiB_2 is also used as vaporization boat or vessel of vacuum-deposited film (like Al, Cu, Cr, Ag, Au, Ge, TiN, etc.). It is also used as a reinforcement particle for Al metal-based composites used in automobile industries, impact resistance cutting tool, crucibles, armor, etc. ZrB_2 is used as the protection tube for continuous temperature measurement in metallurgical industries and the secondary heating electrode of the tundish.

TABLE 12.7   Properties of Some Metal Borides Used in Refractory Industries

Material	Density (g/cm³)	Melting Point (°C)	Thermal Expansion Coefficient (10^{-6}°C⁻¹)	Thermal Conductivity (W/m K)	Knoop Hardness (Kg mm⁻²)	Elastic Modulus (GPa)
TiB_2	4.5	3225	8.1	60–120	2200	54
ZrB_2	6.08	3250	6.9	45–135	1170	35

12.8 SUMMARY

Zircon and zirconia refractories are important for the presence of ZrO_2, which imparts excellent resistances against corrosion, wear, and abrasion. Zircon is a natural mineral that decomposes at high temperatures. But in the presence of certain impurities, it decomposes at much lower temperatures. Hence, the highest application temperature is limited. Zirconia is rarely available in pure form and has polymorphic transformations. It requires stabilizing additives to avoid sudden volume changes with temperature and stabilization. These refractories are mostly used in glass contact areas and iron and steel industries.

Fused cast refractories are manufactured in a different way compared to conventional sintering techniques. As they are shaped from a molten mass, the presence of porosity is very minimum and they have large-sized grains. These impart very high corrosion resistance and are mainly important as liquid contact refractory, mostly in glass industries.

The retainment of heat in a process is mainly done by the insulating refractory. A dense refractory has a higher thermal conductivity, and intentionally small and uniformly distributed pores are created within the refractory mass to reduce the low thermal conductivity. These refractories are used nearly for all the high-temperature industries but mostly as backup lining. Ceramic fibers are also highly insulating in nature and may have different compositions according to the raw materials used. Mainly the composition of the fibers dictates the property developed and the suitable application temperature and environment. Different shapes may be formed using the fibers, as required to prevent heat loss and sealing of the furnaces.

Carbon refractories are made from different natural and synthetic sources of carbon and mostly important for the high thermal conductivity and resistances against thermal shock and corrosion. Oxidation of any carbon bearing material limits its applications.

Silicon carbide is a synthetically prepared material and important for its thermal conductivity, thermal shock, and corrosion resistances. It has greater oxidation resistance than carbon and more widely used compared to carbon refractories.

There are many other non-oxides that are used as an additive to impart certain specific properties in refractory compositions. Among them boron carbide, aluminum nitride, boron nitride, and metal borides are important. All of them are prepared synthetically and are very strongly bonded material. Mostly they are used to impart wear and abrasion resistances.

QUESTIONS AND ASSIGNMENTS

1. Why are zircon and zirconia refractories important? Mention the application areas of these refractories with the reasoning for their applications.

2. Why does zirconia require stabilizing additives? Describe in detail.

3. How are fused cast refractories made?

4. What are the different types of fused cast refractories used?

5. What are the different applications of fused cast refractories?

6. Why are insulation refractories important?

7. Why are small and uniform distribution of pores important for the insulating properties?

8. Why are the insulation refractories not used as hot face lining?

9. How are ceramic fibers made?

10. Describe different classification techniques for ceramic fibers.

11. Why is carbon important as a refractory?

12. What are the different sources of carbon for making refractory? How is a carbon refractory made?

13. What are the application areas of carbon refractories?

14. What are the advantages of silicon carbide as a refractory material?

15. Describe different bonding systems used for silicon carbide refractories.

16. Mention the applications of silicon carbide as a refractory material.

17. What are the different nitrides used in the refractory? Describe any one of them.

18. What are the different borides used in refractory? Write in detail about the metals borides.

BIBLIOGRAPHY

1. *Refractories Handbook*, The Technical Association of Refractories, Tokyo, Japan, 1998.
2. Harbison Walker, *Handbook of Refractory Practice*, Harbison Walker Refractories Co., PA, 2005.

3. B. Brezny and R. Engel, Evaluation of zircon brick for steel ladle slag lines, *American Ceramic Society Bulletin*, 63(7), 880–883, 1984.

4. D. Urffer, The use of zircon in refractories for glass making, *Industrial Minerals*, 344, 49–53, 1996.

5. G. F. Comstock, Some experiments with zircon and zirconia refractories, *Journal of the American Ceramic Society*, 16(1), 12–35, 1933.

6. I. A. Lowe, J. Wosinski, and G. Davis, Stabilizing distressed glass furnace melter crowns, *Ceramic Engineering and Science Proceedings*, 18(1), 164–179, 1997.

7. R. Sarkar and A. Baskey, Decomposition and densification study of zircon with additives, *Interceram*, 60(5), 308–311, 2011.

8. R. L. Bullard, P. C. Cheng, and B. F. J. Schiefer, Long term casting with zirconia nozzles, *Electric Furnace Conference Proceedings*, Vol. 49, pp. 345–354, Toronto, Canada, 12–15 November, 1991.

9. *Standard Classification for Fusion-Cast Refractory Blocks and Shapes*, ASTM Standard C1547-02, 2013.

10. L. J. Manfredo and R. N. McNally, The corrosion resistance of high ZrO_2 fusion-cast Al_2O_3–ZrO_2–SiO_2 glass refractories in soda lime glass, *Journal of Materials Science*, 19(4), 1272–1276, 1984.

11. D. Au, S. Cockcroft, and D. Maijer, Crack defect formation during manufacture of fused cast alumina refractories, *Metallurgical and Materials Transactions A*, 33(7), 2053–2065, 2002.

12. E. Novak, *Refractory Engineering: Materials, Design and Construction*, 2nd edn., Vulkan-Verlag, Essen, 2005.

13. A. Rand, A. S. Ahmed, and V. P. S. Ramos, The role of carbon in refractories, *Tehran International Conference on Refractories*, Tehran, Iran, May 4–6, 2004.

14. A. R. Chesti, *Refractories: Manufacture, Properties and Applications*, Prentice-Hall of India, New Delhi, 1986.

15. E. Mohamed and E. Ewais, Carbon based refractories, *Journal of the Ceramic Society of Japan*, 112(10), 517–532, 2004.

16. J. H. Chesters, *Refractories—Production and Properties*, Woodhead Publishing, Cambridge, UK, 2006.

17. A. L. Shashi Mohan, Silicon carbide refractories: India 2020, *Proceedings of the 8th India International Refractories Congress (IREFCON 10)*, pp. 86–91, Kolkata, India, 2010.

18. A. Lipp, K. A. Schwetz, and K. Hunold, Hexagonal boron nitride: Fabrication, properties, and application, *Journal of the European Ceramic Society*, 5(1), 3–9, 1989.

19. G. Zhang, M. Ando, T. Ohji, and S. Kanzaki, High-performance boron nitride-containing composites by reaction synthesis for the applications in the steel industry, *International Journal of Applied Ceramic Technology*, 2(2), 162–171, 2005.

20. H. Tanaka, Silicon carbide powder and sintered materials, *Journal of the Ceramic Society of Japan*, 119(3), 218–233, 2011.

CHAPTER 13

Unshaped (Monolithic) Refractories

13.1 INTRODUCTION AND ADVANTAGES

Conventionally refractories are considered as industrial products primarily used for any high-temperature processing, especially for the basic industries like iron and steel, glass, cement, non-ferrous metallurgy and foundry, ceramic, and white-wares. Also, it was a traditional concept to consider the refractories as a product with definite shape and size, used to make furnace and kilns for firing. But this conventional concept was not true as a good amount of refractories are unshaped in nature. Unshaped refractory is not a new material. Probably it was used along with the shaped refractory initially. Placing and fixing of any refractory shapes essentially require mortars that belong to the unshaped refractory. Any repair work used for refractory lining is essentially an unshaped refractory or uses the concept of unshaped refractory. But in early days, it was not considered and recorded as a separate class of refractory, as unshaped refractory, as being considered today.

The first well-recorded information on unshaped refractory is available from literature. In 1856, H. S. C. Devile prepared a refractory crucible using a refractory concrete based on alumina aggregate and alumina cement. Plastic refractory was first commercialized by W. A. L. Schaeffer in 1914. Schaeffer founded a company, originally named Pliable Brick Company, which was later changed to Plibrico Company LLC, which started the business of making unshaped refractory. Schaeffer recognized the fact that refractory lining for various industries will become complicated as a simple shape would not be sufficient for lining them. If we look into the recorded history of unshaped refractory, then plastic refractory was started in 1914, followed by the castable refractory. The first information on castable is available as a patent, filed in 1923, where alumina–silica–zirconia system was shaped by simple casting technique and then fused to densify. Next comes the gunning mass, which was patented (filed) in 1951 for a silica-based patching mass using a spray gun. Then in the 1970s, deflocculated castable system was developed that can be cast in the molds using vibration at a lower water requirements. Next comes the self-flowing castables in 1987, where low cement castable composition was reported in Japan to flow under its own weight. This was followed by shotcreteing materials in 1989, which were used first in Japan to coat a refractory surface.

Unshaped refractories (also called monolithic refractories) are unfired products and do not have any definite shape and dimensions. They can have similar chemical properties and may show similar or better physical, mechanical, thermomechanical, and other refractory related properties than the shaped ones. The term "monolithic" comes from two different Latin words, namely *mono* meaning "single" and *lithus* meaning "structure." So monolithics are refractories that can make a refractory lining with a single structure, that is, without any joint.

A shaped refractory is a prefered one with a definite and specific shape and dimensions and having a homogeneous structure and properties, whereas an unshaped refractory is a mixture of graded refractory aggregates and fines homogeneously mixed with bond materials and property-enhancing additives, mixed in a predetermined fixed ratio. They are packed as loose materials and transferred to the user industries where mixing (in most cases) with a fixed amount of liquid (commonly water) is done using intensive mixers and installed by special application techniques. As per international standard ISO 1927 (5) and European standard EN 1402-1, monolithics are defined as "mixtures which consist of an aggregate and a bond or bonds, prepared ready for use either directly in the condition in which they are supplied or after the addition of one or more suitable liquids, and which satisfy the requirements of refractories."

The main advantages of unshaped refractories are as follows:

1. It involves no shaping and no firing, hence manufacturing of these materials are easier, less process dependent, less polluting, and economic.

2. Any shape and any dimension of the refractory lining can be fabricated, which is not possible in shaped products. Any complicated shape with as many curvatures, slopes, and contours and large dimensions can be made by unshaped refractories, which are not possible by the shaping processes, such as pressing and extrusion.

3. As the number of joints is less or jointless (or without joint), unshaped refractories have much greater corrosion and wear resistance compared to shaped and bricks as the joints are a weak point to corrode and wear away.

4. Installation of conventionally shaped refractory lining is a skilled job for a prolonged time, whereas unshaped refractory placement is simple, less skilled, and quick. Thus, installation process is also economic.

5. Unshaped refractory can bond with itself easily, even with a fired lining. Thus, when a lining is worn away due to use, the lost lining can be filled by the fresh material with similar composition and fired, and the whole lining can act as afresh. But for brick lining, when it is worn sufficiently, the lining has to be dismantled, and rest of the brick has to be thrown away, and a completely new lining is required to be done. Thus, nearly half of the brick remains unutilized and relining is also a time-consuming and costly affair.

Due to these various advantages, the unshaped refractory has replaced the shaped ones in a big way. Mostly in the advanced countries, the use of unshaped refractory is more than 50% of the total refractory. But in developing and underdeveloped countries, their usage is very low, mainly due to difficulties in certain process automation, control on installation and application techniques, and for control on the high-temperature processing at the user industry.

13.2 CLASSIFICATION

From the major constituent point of view, unshaped refractories are mostly based on alumina and aluminosilicate materials. Basic unshaped refractories are used but only for certain special applications and with specific application techniques. Silica-based unshaped is also very limited. Carbon-containing unshaped refractories are also available but with a very limited amount of carbon. Carbon is hydrophobic in nature and it does not disperse well in aqueous medium. So non-aqueous liquid is essential to disperse carbon, which are generally highly viscous in nature.

Again as the unshaped refractories are not compacted (only shape is given by different techniques), special binders are required for strength development both at ambient and high temperatures and also to retain the shape at low temperatures. There are different bonding materials and classification is also done based on these bonding materials present in the unshaped refractory, like cement-bonded and gel-bonded materials, but they are not a major classification of unshaped refractory and generally used as subclassifications.

Generally, the classification of unshaped refractories is based on the application techniques, and unshaped refractories are popular as per the application method used for installation. To cope up with a specific application, sometimes special additives are added and also the properties may vary according to the installation methods. Table 13.1 provides details about such classification.

TABLE 13.1　Application Techniques and the Corresponding Names of the Unshaped Refractories

Application Technique	Name of Refractory	Description
Casting/pouring	Castable	A dry mix of different sized materials mixed with liquid (water) at the application site. Installation is done by simple pouring method in a gap space, made by using a former, where the lining is to be done, with or without vibration.
Ramming	Ramming mass	Granular material contains lesser fines than castable, placed by ramming methods like hand or pneumatic ramming, and shovel tamping. It is mostly done at the bottom surface and rammed material thickness is kept below 100–150 mm.
Gunning	Gunning mass	A dry mix of different fractions finer than castable. The dry mix needs to flow under pneumatic pressure through a hose pipe of gunning equipment from the stock hopper and mix with liquid (water) at application nozzle.
Pasting	Plastic/pliable/patching mass	It is not a dry mass rather a ready-to-use material, supplied as a premixed condition with liquid. Consistency and quality of the material vary with the specific application method. Small repair is done (like cracks) but also used for greater area repair by mallet hitting or pneumatic rammers.
Spaying/shotcreting	Spray mass/shotcrete	These are sprayable refractory, similar to gunning in character but with finer sizes. Shotcrete is a further advanced form for better application and performance of the lining.
Vibration (dry)	Dry vibratable mass	Dry premixed mass generally contains thermosetting binders, are applied with vibration to enhance the compaction and sets and hardens when heated.

13.3 SPECIAL RAW MATERIALS AND ADDITIVES

Among all the different types of unshaped refractories, the major constituent is mainly alumina and alumina-silicates and in some limited cases, it is magnesia or silica. Detailed discussion on the commercially available and widely used raw materials for alumina has been done in Section 6.2 and for magnesia in Section 8.2. Mostly these materials constitute the major portion of the different unshaped refractories. Other than these, matrix modifiers are added, which are not used in shaped refractories. Matrix modifiers are part of the major constituent materials and are always in fine fractions and essentially required for the betterment of the properties. Other than the major constituent, there are different other essential components required to make an unshaped refractory. These can be classified as binders and property-enhancing additives, which are detailed in the following.

13.3.1 Fines of Major Constituents

Unshaped refractories widely differ from shaped refractories as they are not compacted during the shaping (shaping during installation without any load) and so sintering is weak in these compositions. Also the concept of packing used for unshaped refractories is never to attain the most dense structure because they need to move, either flow or transported, during application or installation and highest packing (compaction) will restrict this behavior. Hence the sintering in the composition during firing will be limited due to this less packed conditions, which may result in poor densification and strength in the final product. These problems are somewhat taken care by addition of special fine fractions of the major constituents with special characteristics. These fine fractions need to help the flow properties and also to improve the sintering and strength development. Thus these fines modify the matrix part of the unshaped refractory and are called matrix modifiers. For alumina sources, some special types of property tailored alumina fines, which are generally not used in shaped refractories, are used in unshaped refractories to modify the matrix so that both the requirements can be met. These special aluminas are technical alumina fines and reactive alumina. Fineness and shapes of these fines are important. Again the particle size distribution is tailored, by using bimodal or multimodal distribution, so that they can improve the compaction of the whole composition. These alumina fines are essential for the matrix phase in technologically improved unshaped refractories. But for very conventional unshaped refractories, these matrix modifiers are not used mainly due to their high cost.

13.3.2 Binder

Binders are essential for the development of strength at the ambient and elevated temperatures and also to retain the shape at green conditions as no compaction is involved in the shaping process during installations of unshaped refractories. Also binders help to sinter the compositions, as there is no compaction during shaping and mass transfer for sintering is less, resulting in poor densification and strength. Initially plastic clay was used as a binder for an unshaped refractory. The plastic nature helped to retain the shape, stickiness provided the strength at low temperatures, and fine size improved the densification behaviour. But higher water requirement, shrinkage, poor strength, and poor hot properties were the associated drawbacks. Then came the alumina-containing cement. During the initial days, the alumina content of the refractory cement was less than 50% and the quality and properties along with the alumina content were improved significantly with time. But presence of lime in the composition resulted in poor high temperature properties and refractory researchers, manufacturers, and users were looking for a binder without lime. Then came the cement-free bonding systems, like sol-gel, hydrated alumina, and phosphates. But all the different bonding systems have certain limitations and are used in a limited manner. And still today, high alumina cement is used as the major bonding material for unshaped refractories.

13.3.2.1 High Alumina Cement

At the very beginning of unshaped refractories, people thought of using ordinary portland cement (OPC) as a binder for unshaped refractory due to the similarity of the material with concretes. But OPC has about 60%–65% of CaO, which is deadly for the refractory industries. Also due to dehydration of the bond, the structure will collapse above ~625°C and in the cyclic condition above even 400°C. So OPC is never used as a bond in unshaped refractory.

Alumina-based cement was first patented by Lafarge in 1908 in France, and first commercial production was also started by Lafarge in 1913. But originally alumina cement was developed and used for construction industries due to its better corrosion resistance than OPC. The use of alumina cement for high-temperature applications started in the mid-1920s, both in the United States and France, when calcined clay and crushed fireclay bricks were mixed with bauxite-based alumina cement. But these materials were of very low grade due to poor mixing and application technique.

In the initial days, use of cement was high at ~12–18 wt% and so the water requirement (for cement hydration and flow) was also very high at about 10–20 wt%. During firing, the hydraulic bond of cement particles breaks due to dehydration, removal of moisture occurs, resulting in porous and very weak structures. So high density and strength were difficult to attain without the formation of liquid phase. Also a high amount of lime in cement easily reacts with the alumina and aluminosilicate fines and forms the liquid phases at a much lower temperature. Hence, these unshaped compositions were only applicable for low temperatures.

As the operating temperatures of the refractory user industries, especially the metallurgical sector, are increasing due to greater purity of their products, high temperature withstanding refractories are in demand and unshaped refractories with reduced cement content were being tried since long. In 1969, the first patent was filed in France for the low cement-containing composition wherein the cement was reduced to 4–6 wt% with near equal amount of water demand by using some flow-modifying additives, namely silica fume and dispersants. Fine silica fume particles improves the flow and improves packing as was done by cement and cement hydrates. This development has increased the application temperature from 1300–1350°C level to 1500–1550°C level. Further reduction improvement in cement content continued by further controlling the aggregates and their granulometry, quality of cements, and use of additives.

The alumina cement can be of different grades depending on the alumina content and accordingly their raw materials, properties, and application areas change. Low alumina-containing cements, initially developed, are still in use and are prepared from lime stone and bauxite. Impurities of these raw materials remain within the cement composition and limits its highest application temperature to 1250–1300°C. The purer variety of natural raw materials marginally improves the properties and the application temperatures. Pure variety of alumina cements are prepared mainly from synthetic raw materials, namely, hydrated lime (produced by hydration of calcined lime stone) and calcined alumina (from Bayer's process). These cements can have very high alumina content, even upto 80 wt% Al_2O_3, with very minimum amount of impurity. They are commonly referred as high alumina cement (HAC).

$CaO–Al_2O_3$ phase diagram is shown in Figure 13.1. The two major and desirable phases present in purer variety of HAC are monocalcium aluminate ($CaO \cdot Al_2O_3$, CA), the principal reactive phase that hydrates and provides bond, and calcium dialuminate ($CaO \cdot 2Al_2O_3$, CA_2), the secondary hydraulic phase (poor hydration activity). There may be some unwanted phases also like, dodeca-calcium hepta-aluminate ($12CaO \cdot 7Al_2O_3$), which is flash setting in character, and calcium hexa-aluminate ($CaO \cdot 6Al_2O_3$), which is non-hydraulic in nature. The details of the CaO–Al_2O_3 system is given in Figure 13.1. The presence of $3CaO \cdot Al_2O_3$ (less likely to be present due to wide compositional difference) and $12CaO \cdot 7Al_2O_3$ makes the cement very fast setting, or flash setting, due to very high amount of lime, whereas $CaO \cdot 6Al_2O_3$ makes it non-hydraulic. In impure cement system, there are some non-hydraulic impurity phases also like gehlenite ($2CaO \cdot Al_2O_3 \cdot SiO_2$), calcium titanate ($CaO \cdot TiO_2$), calcium ferrite ($CaO \cdot Fe_2O_3$), and tetracalcium alumino ferrite ($4CaO \cdot Al_2O_3 \cdot Fe_2O_3$). Table 13.2 shows the hydration scheme of the two hydraulic phases of calcium aluminate.

Metastable hydroxide CAH_{10} and C_2AH_8 phases convert to stable C_3AH_6 phase during curing and drying of the unshaped refractory after shaping. During drying and firing of the product, all the CAH_{10} and C_2AH_8 phases are completely converted into the C_3AH_6 phase below 200°C and on further heating at ~300°C, it is converted to anhydrous metastable $C_{12}A_7$

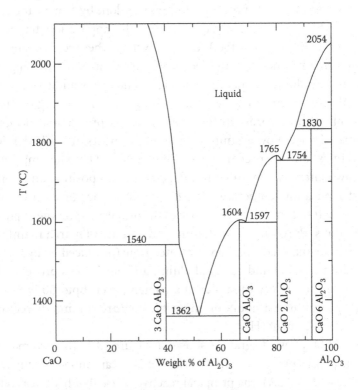

FIGURE 13.1 Phase diagram of CaO–Al_2O_3 system.

TABLE 13.2   Hydration Reaction of Two Major Calcium Aluminate Phases

Temperature	Hydration Reaction for	
	For CA	For CA_2
<18°C	$CA + 10H = CAH_{10}$	$CA_2 + 13H = CAH_{10} + AH_3$
Between 18°C and 30°C	$2CA + 11 H = C_2AH_8 + AH_3$	$2CA_2 + 17H = C_2AH_8 + 3AH_3$
>30°C	$3CA + 12H = C_3AH_6 + 2AH_3$	$3CA_2 + 21H = C_3AH_6 + 5AH_3$
Final changes (depends on time, humidity, and temperature)	$2CAH_{10} = C_2AH_8 + AH_3 + 9H$ $3C_2AH_8 = 2C_3AH_6 + AH_3 + 9H$	

Note: $C = CaO$, $A = Al_2O_3$, and $H = H_2O$.

phase. Again on further heating between 900°C and 1000°C, $C_{12}A_7$ reacts with finer alumina particles in the matrix phase and is converted into CA phase. Due to dehydration and hydraulic bond breaking activity, there is a drastic fall in the strength of the cement containing unshaped refractories above 300°C and the fall is stronger when the cement content is higher. This reduced strength remains till sintering is started above 1000°C.

The amount of water used in making the unshaped refractory plays an important role in the development of property. Water is required for hydration of cement particles and also for flow consistency of the material. Any excess of water will cause a void space in the structure and will result in reduced density and strength. Again excess water helps to grow the cement hydrate particles, resulting in bigger-sized hydrate crystals, bigger-sized pores among them, and poor strength properties.

Again when the cement contains predominantly the CA_2 phase, the amount of lime is less and the cement will have reduced hydraulic activity. But there are techniques like increased fineness and increased reactivity of CA_2 phases by controlling grain growth, etc., by which the hydration tendency can be improved. Again the presence of higher alumina CA_2 results in an excess formation of AH_3, which fills the porous structure of the unshaped refractory in a better way, resulting in improved compaction and strength values. Also the CA_2 phase has a decomposition temperature about 160°C higher compared to that of the CA phase (Figure 13.1). So the CA_2 phase containing HAC is better in higher temperature properties.

13.3.2.2 Colloidal Silica

The use of calcium aluminate cement results in relatively poor high-temperature properties due to formation of low melting phases. For high cement containing compositions, the total CaO present is high enough that reacts with the impurity phases and forms low melting compounds in the $CaO-Al_2O_3-Fe_2O_3$ and $CaO-Al_2O_3$ SiO_2 systems. A reduction in cement content reduced the amount of CaO considerably, which may result in reduced room temperature strength, fines content, and flow character. The addition of other fine materials like silica fume improves certain properties but may affect the high-temperature properties by forming liquid phases, mainly in the $CaO-Al_2O_3$ SiO_2 systems. Also corrosion resistance of lime-containing system was not the best. Curing and dewatering steps also require special attention to avoid any explosion, spalling, and cracking. Hence the researchers were in search of CaO free bond systems.

Among different lime-free bonds, colloidal silica, or silica sol bonding has got wide popularity and commercial success. Colloidal silica is a stable dispersion of silica particles in a liquid, usually water, where particles are small enough and suspended that they don't settle but large enough that they do not pass through a membrane but allow other molecules and ions to pass freely. Colloidal silica is denser than water due to presence of silica particles and electrostatically stabilized to form stable suspension. The basic units of colloidal silica are $[SiO_4]^{4-}$ tetrahedra, which are randomly distributed, resulting in an amorphous nature of the material.

It is prepared in a multistep process. An alkali–silicate (sodium silicate) solution is first neutralized to form a silica nuclei, which are usually just a few nanometers in diameter. Polymerization of these nuclei starts without the alkali ions, when the stability of the sol is disturbed by change in pH and temperature. Thus the sol particles grow in size. So to maintain the stable sol character, a control on pH and temperature is essential and generally the sols are stored between 5°C and 30°C. At very low temperatures, the sol loses its stability and precipitates out as a silica particle. Again at elevated temperatures, the growth of the particles increases and thus decreases the long-term stability of the silica sol. Other than the refractory applications, colloidal silica is also important for manufacturing of coatings, catalysts, paper industries, and moisture absorbents.

The use of silica sol replacing alumina cement is a great improvement in unshaped refractories and resulted in improved high-temperature properties. The principle behind this bonding is the formation of a "gel" from "sol," which surrounds and encapsulates the refractory aggregates through a three-dimensional skeleton network. During drying, the hydroxyl groups (Si–OH) of the sol on the surface of the particles are convert into siloxane bonds (Si–O–Si) due to the removal of moisture and forms the rigid three-dimensional network. This gelation can also be induced by water removal, pH variations, and using additives called gelling agents.

This gelled network around the refractory particles provides strength to the system after drying. After removal of the moisture, the structure is highly permeable and allows easy removal of moisture from the unshaped refractory, reducing cracks and explosive spalling. On further heating, the fine gel particles help in sintering by forming ceramic bonding at a lower temperature. Also silica sol helps in flowability due to its fine size and spherical shape. The formation of mullite on firing in alumina-based compositions also helps in improving the corrosion resistance and the high-temperature properties of the unshaped refractories.

The advantages of colloidal silica over high alumina cement are listed as follows:

1. Less mixing time due to absence of additives.

2. Higher viscosity (than water) improves separation between the refractory particles that improves flowability.

3. Reduced drying time and drying defects due to the absence of free water for mixing and permeable structure.

4. Inherent formation of mullite in alumina compositions improves corrosion resistance and hot strength properties.

5. Better high-temperature properties due to absence low melting compounds in $CaO–Al_2O_3–Fe_2O_3$ and $CaO–Al_2O_3–SiO_2$ systems.

6. Better high-temperature properties result in longer campaign life and reduced downtime of operation.

7. Longer shelf-life due to the absence of any hygroscopic phases.

8. Fine silica particles from the sol coat the non-oxides in a better way, resulting in improved oxidation resistance and better performance for non-oxide-containing compositions.

13.3.2.3 Hydratable Alumina

Hydratable alumina binders are increasingly used in no cement-unshaped refractories for its unique character. In this bonding, an inert matrix containing alumina formed from hydratable alumina binder can provide a non-reactive protective border surrounding alumina aggregates. Thus, a complete alumina system, having both the aggregate and matrix as alumina, without any secondary phase can be developed that will have improved slag resistance, fracture toughness, hot strength and resistance against thermal shock, abrasion, and erosion. The absence of lime and other impurities nearly nullify the formation of any low melting compounds, and high strength develops due to the ceramic bond formation at high temperatures.

Hydratable aluminas are low-crystalline mesophase transition aluminas generally produced by vacuum calcinations (~550–600°C) or flash calcination (between 600°C and 900°C) of gibbsite, resulting mainly in a high-surface area transition phase, called rho-alumina. The bonding character of rho-alumina develops from its rehydration behavior when the same is in contact with moisture (or water vapor). The hydration reaction is as follows:

$$\text{rho-Al}_2O_3 + H_2O \rightarrow Al_2O_3 \cdot 3H_2O + Al_2O_3 \cdot (1 \rightarrow 2)H_2O$$

A thick layer of gel is formed during hydration, which subsequently crystallizes partly to bayerite and boehmite phases and the rest remaining as an amorphous gel. The amount of these gels formed depends on the hydration temperature and pH. Interlocking bayerite crystals and the gel fill the pores and the interfacial defects and form a honeycomb-type structure on the refractory aggregates that provides green strength. Such crystallization also favors the formation of crystals on the surface of the aggregates, connecting adjacent grains to the surrounding matrix. During heating, the hydrated phases lose their chemical water, are converted to stable α-Al_2O_3 fine particles, which at higher temperatures help in sintering. However, hydratable aluminas have a few limitations, like they are highly susceptible to explosive spalling during drying due to less permeable structure and also the development of strength at low temperatures are poor. Economically hydratable alumina is also not favorable.

13.3.2.4 Phosphates

Phosphate-bonded refractories are known since 1950s but wide commercial application started too late. This category comes under the broad classification of chemical-bonded refractories where phosphate acts as a chemical bond. Another important chemical bond used for refractories is sodium silicate, but due to its low melting point, it is used in very limited cases. Phosphate bonding is typically used for "plastic" refractories and as it has no lime, it does not set easily at ambient conditions. Freedom from setting allows it to remain as a moistened condition for nearly indefinite time periods and allows great working time for the lining or repair. But it is used in limited cases due to its poor strength development. Poor strength, poor resistance against corrosion, and wear for phosphate-bonded materials are due to relatively weak and porous structure coming from higher liquid content for installation and application. In contrast to cement-bonded compositions, which develop strength in basic conditions, phosphates work better in acidic atmosphere. The bond is developed in a unshaped refractory by addition or in situ generation of phosphates, either by reaction of phosphoric acid (H_3PO_4) with metal oxides (say alumina) or by addition of phosphates directly like mono-aluminum phosphate [MAP or $Al(H_2PO_4)_3$].

When the first option is used, the phosphoric acid (H_3PO_4) solution initially reacts with Al_2O_3 (above 127°C upto 427°C) or with $Al(OH)_3$ (at room temperature) forming monoaluminum phosphate (MAP) $Al(H_2PO_4)_3$. This MAP decomposes on heating to form ortho-aluminum phosphate (OAP) till 1327°C and which, on further heating, forms pure alumina and phosphoric pentoxide in the gaseous state.

$$6H_3PO_4 + Al_2O_3 = 2Al(H_2PO_4)_3 + 3H_2O \text{ (temperature 127–427°C)}$$

$$3H_3PO_4 + Al(OH)_3 = Al(H_2PO_4)_3 + 3H_2O \text{ (room temperature)}$$

$$Al(H_2PO_4)_3 = AlPO_4 + 3H_2O + P_2O_5 \text{ (temperature 732–1327°C)}$$

$$2AlPO_4 = Al_2O_3 + P_2O_5 \text{ (above 1350°C)}$$

So this bonding finally results in pure alumina with no trace of phosphorus in the fired composition. Hence it produces no secondary phases. But there are several disadvantages associated with phosphates. Primarily the setting of the material is very slow and sluggish. In order to speed up the reaction, setting agents are used like MgO, CaO, calcium aluminates, and so on. These additives induce an acid–base reaction, forming amorphous to crystalline phosphates that enhance the refractory hardening and other properties. Also phosphate bonding requires a considerable amount of mechanical moisture for workability and so a long heat-up schedule is required for drying. Again the green strength is weak due to lack of strong bonding, like in cement. On firing, the bond system loses a considerable amount of strength at operating temperatures above 1300°C till ceramic bond forms on sintering. This binder system has also poor ability to bond with existing fired refractories. In addition, a high chance of lamination exists in the refractory lining, as they have weak bonding strength.

In the second type of bonding, dry phosphates are used with water. The most commonly available and used phosphate powder is MAP due to its high solubility in water, greater bonding strength, and reaction with basic and amphoteric raw materials at low temperatures. The performance of this bonding depends on the size of the phosphate powders, mixing process of dry phosphate with the refractory aggregate, and dissolution of phosphates in water and its reaction. This type of phosphate bond gives reasonably quick set times and moderate green strengths due to the reaction of the dry phosphate and water. A proper heat-up schedule is required to remove moisture and to avoid cracking and spalling. Again improper mixing and dissolution of phosphate will result in inconsistent bonding and properties of the unshaped refractory.

Phosphate bonding is used for alumina-based compositions but not used for silica or magnesia compositions. Silica does not react with phosphoric acid at low temperatures but forms $SiO_2 \cdot P_2O_5$ and $2SiO_2 \cdot P_2O_5$ compounds at high temperatures, which are low melting (1100–1300°C) compounds. For magnesia, the phosphoric acid reacts instantly and setting of phosphate is very fast. Also different magnesium phosphates are formed, and all are low melting compounds, maximum being newbeyrite ($MgHPO_4 \cdot 3H_2O$) with a melting point of 1327°C. Hence, phosphate bonding is avoided in silica and basic systems.

13.3.3 Silica Fume (Flow Modifier)

The concept of unshaped refractory, especially the castables, has been changed with the reduction in cement content, which was only possible by using the flow modifier, silica fume. The use of silica fume has reduced the amount of cement from about 12–20 wt% level to 4–6 wt% level and improved the high-temperature properties without affecting the installation and low temperature properties. Silica fume, also known as micro silica, is a by-product of silicon and ferro-silicon industries. It is a noncrystalline polymorph of silica having average size of particles below 0.15 micron, surface area 20 m²/g, and spherical in shape. The main application area of silica fume is high-performance concrete, since about 1950s, for improvement of flowability due to its shape, size, and pozzolanic activity. As this silica fume consists of minimum 90% silica, which is a good refractory material, the use of silica fume in refractory was planned.

Silica fume enhances the flowability of the unshaped refractory as similar to the concrete, mainly due to its spherical shape and finer size. Thus it helps in reduction in water content, which is otherwise essentially required to get flow and movement in the refractory mass. Also finer-sized silica fume particles easily enter in the voids, even very small in size and fill them, thus enhancing the packing of the refractory, densification, sintering, and helps in strength development. They are also termed as microfiller. Hence, the presence of silica fume reduces the requirement of the cement and its hydrate phases to fill the voids and packing, and thus a reduction in cement content is possible. Also silica fume has some pozzolanic activity, reacts with water to form hydrated bond, mainly in the $CaO-SiO_2-H_2O$ and $CaO-SiO_2-Al_2O_3-H_2O$ systems. Also during the formation process, some negative charge remains on the surface of silica fumes, which help to disperse the cement-containing systems, where cement particles are positive in charge. Thus they also reduce the water requirement by satisfying the charge of the cement particles. Being a major source of silica in high alumina compositions, silica fume also helps in the formation of mullite at high temperatures, which enhances hot strength, corrosion, and thermal shock resistances.

Typically, a commercial silica fume contains silica in the range 90%–95% but the major impurities present are carbon, in the range of 0.2%–1.5% (coming from the silicon and ferrosilicon industry, used as raw material for carbothermal reduction), iron oxide in the range of up to 2%, alkali oxides (Na_2O and K_2O) up to 4%, alkaline earth oxide (CaO and MgO) up to 3%, and alumina up to 1%. Impurities are harmful in the performance of silica fume as a refractory material. Also, higher content of alkalis affect the setting behavior, and it enhances the setting of the unshaped refractory allowing less working time.

13.3.4 Dispersants and Antisetting Agents

These are the additives especially required for the cement-containing compositions where flowability is an important parameter like low cement and advanced castables. They work on the conventional deflocculation theory of increasing double layer thickness, thus increasing the charge stabilization of the matrix system and increasing flow properties. Dispersant-containing matrix acts as a deflocculated particulate system that allows the whole unshaped refractory including the coarse aggregates to flow. The dispersants contain polar molecules that get absorbed by the particles, and they increase the surface charge. Thus, a surface repulsion occurs, resulting in a decrease in viscosity and a stable, flowable matrix system is developed. Also, the dispersants increase the pH range of the matrix stabilization. The use of organic polymer compounds as dispersants with high polymerization (large molecular size) also helps in increasing the double layer thickness at a lower concentration and results in better deflocculation. The common inorganic dispersants are pyrophosphates $[(P_2O_7)^{-4}]$, tripolyphosphate $[(P_3O_{10})^{-5}]$, and hexa-metaphosphate $[(P_6O_{18})^{-6}]$ and common organic dispersants are citrates, polyacrylates, and polymethacrylates.

Antisetting agents are additives, especially added to cement-containing compositions, which delay the setting of cements. The addition of water in an unshaped refractory will initiate the hydration of cement and the cement will start setting. As the mixing of unshaped refractory with liquid is difficult at the exact location of application, a time gap between addition of water (liquid) and setting is required for transporting the mixed mass and installation of the material, which is technically called as working time. So these antisetting agents provide that working time and keep the mixed mass workable and flowable even after addition of water for some fixed time period. Antisetting agents are generally hygroscopic in nature. They absorb the moisture added to the unshaped refractory and delay the cement hydration reactions. But with time, cement particles draw out the moisture from these hygroscopic materials and starts to hydrate and then set. This time delay is essential for better flow, placement and installation, and final properties of the refractory. But higher addition of antisetting agent will delay the setting of cement for a long time, resulting in poor or no setting, flow out or deformation of unshaped refractory, poor strength, and other properties. Hence the amount of antisetting agent is very crucial for proper installation and property development of cement containing unshaped refractories. The common antisetting agents used are citric acid, oxalic acids, and tartaric acids and their ammonium and sodium salts.

13.3.5 Fibers

Unshaped refractories are added with different fibers for imparting some special character required for final property development. They are as follows.

13.3.5.1 Organic Fiber

When the unshaped refractory is cast, the water added performs mainly two functions. One is for the hydration reaction and initial strength development and also as water for free movement or flow. This loose free water comes out from the surface during drying of the shape. Now during drying, as the heating is done from the outside, the surface gets dried and drying shrinkage is strong at the surface only, resulting in reduced passage for the interior moisture vapor to come out from the surface of the shape. But at the drying temperature, the water is vaporised, a huge internal vapor pressure is created within the shape. This pressure, if higher than the dried or green strength of the product, the shape will crack, break, or shatter. This drying breakage is termed as explosive spalling during drying.

To avoid this problem, organic fibers are added to the refractory compositions that will melt and create a small passage for the removal of the water vapor during drying. Hence, these organic fibers are essentially needed to melt and evaporate out from the composition before the formation of pressurized moisture vapor and need to be very thin in diameter. Hence, organic fibers of polyethylene (melting point ~120°C) and polystyrene (melting point ~165°C) are used. These fibers have a high aspect ratio, with dimensions of 6–10 mm long and ~10–30 micron in diameter and are used in the range of 0.02–0.1 wt%. The use of these fibers creates a channel in the unshaped refractory, helps the vapor to go out and nullifies explosive spalling, and allows higher heating rate for drying and firing of the unshaped refractory.

13.3.5.2 Metallic Fiber

These fibers are mostly chromium- and nickel-containing steel alloy, have high melting and deformation temperature, prepared by wire drawn, centrifuged out from the melt, milled from the block, etc. methods, used to impart some tensile character in the unshaped refractories. The fibers are about 20–30 mm long, 0.3–0.4 mm in diameter and used in the range of 3–6 wt% in the unshaped refractory. These fibers are added to such compositions that are applied to thermal shock-prone areas. The fibers allow the refractory mass to remain in the structure even after cracking due to thermal shock by pinning effect. Thus, they can enhance the life and performance of the refractory. But the addition of metallic fibers affects the flow behavior, increases water demand but improves strength and thermal shock properties. Though these fibers have oxidation resistance till ~1200°C, as they remain within the unshaped refractory and not exactly exposed at the hot surface, they can be used for processes of much higher temperatures.

13.4 BRIEF DETAILS OF DIFFERENT UNSHAPED REFRACTORIES

13.4.1 Castables

Castables are the most studied and commercially most widely used material among the different monolithic refractories. Starting with the development of calcium aluminate cement, refractory castables have progressed from simple mixes of different fractions of main constituents and binder to a complex and technical formulations, suitable for various critical applications with very specific and tailored properties. Shaped refractories are increasingly being replaced by castables in many applications due to the enhanced performance and ease of installation. In general, castables may be defined as blended mixes of different fractions of main constituent with bonding agent and various additives, supplied in dried conditions as loose powders and mixed with a liquid (water) at the user industry and vibrated, poured, pumped, or pneumatically shot into place to form the desired shape or structure that becomes rigid because of hydraulic or chemical setting and then fired to complete the process.

Castables can be of different types depending on the

1. Main constituent (alumina, magnesia, silica, etc.)

2. Amount or percentage of the main constituent (60% alumina, 70% alumina, 90% alumina, etc.)

3. Density (dense, insulating)

4. Bonding material (cement, sol, phosphate, etc.)

5. Amount of bond, especially for cement containing one (conventional cement, low cement, ultralow cement, no cement, etc.)

6. Flow and placement conditions (vibrating, self-flowing, etc.)

Castables have, unlike shaped refractory, a continuous bonding or matrix phase wherein the aggregates are distributed. Hence, development of matrix phase is critical for the performance of the castables. So fines and additives play the major role in the property development and performance of the castables. Also, contrary to shaped refractories, castables need to flow with density and strength achievements. Again density and strength development depends on the compaction among the particles. But increased compaction means rigid structure, greater friction between the particle and reduced flow properties. So two parameters, flow and compaction, are contradictory in nature. So conventional particle packing models, namely discrete models, are not applicable for castable developments, and continuous particle size distribution models are used. This is important for the advanced high-performance castables where a reduction in water demand is a prime factor for better performance. However, for conventional castables, discrete model with wide size distribution of aggregates are used to make the system and process simpler.

Bonding material used and its amount greatly affects the properties and the performance of the castables. For cement-containing compositions, the amount of cement used and its associate additives play a great role in the placement and property development of the castable. Conventional cement castables, containing cement above 12 wt%, require a higher amount of water and results in a porous structure. Also, they have a greater strength in cold conditions due to a greater extent of hydrated phases present but at high temperatures, the formation of liquid phase due to a higher amount of CaO present in combination with alumina and other impurities like SiO_2 and Fe_2O_3 reduce the heat strength and all the high-temperature properties. Also, the decomposition of hydrated phases result in drastic deterioration of the strength at the intermediate temperatures (300–1000°C) till sintering occurs, and a ceramic bond develops. Low cement castables, having cement in the range of 4–6 wt% with fume silica of a similar amount, have improved the properties at high temperatures but still the formation of liquid phases remains, and castables are applicable up to 1550°C. Above this temperature, the formation of low melting compounds, namely, anorthite ($CaO \cdot Al_2O_3 \cdot 2SiO_2$) and gehlenite ($2CaO \cdot Al_2O_3 \cdot SiO_2$), are high and high-temperature properties degrade drastically. The replacement of silica fume by reactive aluminas provides similar flow properties and improves the hot properties of the castables. A further reduction in cement to 1–1.5 wt% makes ultralow cement castables, which further improves the properties by reducing the amount of liquid phase formation. Cement-free compositions are developed to avoid the lime-containing liquid phases. Also the presence of lime in cement-containing compositions adversely affects corrosion resistance. The use of silica sol makes castable with further better hot properties, especially due to inherent mullite phase formation in high-alumina compositions. But, weak coagulation bonding of the silica sol results in poor strength at ambient temperatures. Also, there is no degradation in strength at the intermediate temperatures for sol-containing compositions and high-temperature strength is considerably improved compared to any cement-bonded material. Hydrated alumina-bonded refractories are special kind of material where the whole composition, aggregate and matrix part, can be made of alumina only (for high-alumina compositions) and may result in excellent high-temperature properties, including corrosion resistance. But weak bonding at low temperatures, huge amount of moisture loss (chances of cracking during drying), and poor sintering properties are the difficulties encountered in the attempt to achieve the desired properties. Phosphate-bonded materials are excellent from workability point of view but are porous in character and have weak bonding strength at low temperatures.

The flow characteristic of the castables is important as a better flowing material can easily and accurately achieve the desired shape with intricate design. But excessive high flowability may result in very low viscous material, which may cause separation of aggregate and matrix parts. Poorly flowable mass is difficult to cast resulting in poor placement, installation, and final properties. External energy is supplied using vibration in most of the castables that allow the mixed composition to flow properly and take the intricacies of the shapes. Also there are castable formulations that attain the desired flowability without any external vibration (flows under its weight are called self-flow castable, where precise control of particle size and its distribution are very important). Flowability of the castable mix is important for the initial period (after mixing with water), and then it must decrease gradually with time as the material has to set (harden) and strength development occurs.

Among the properties, density and porosity values depend on how better the voids are filled and how well the composition is densified. In both the cases, fines and the matrix part play an important role. Density also increases with the increase in alumina content of the composition. Thermal conductivity, abrasion resistance, and other properties of the castable increase with an increase in compaction and alumina content. Also, higher room temperature strength will result in better abrasion resistance. However at high temperatures, the abrasion resistance depends on the alumina content and the strength of the bond at those temperatures. Most of the high-temperature properties are dependent on the presence of liquid phase and densification or sintering of the composition.

13.4.2 Ramming Mass

Ramming masses are unshaped refractory, mainly used for installation and repair work and are a granular mass with semiwet or dry consistency. These refractories were very popular when the advanced castable was not developed. But with the development and advancement of low cement, ultralow cement, and sol bonded castables, use of ramming masses have decreased gradually. Ramming mass is mostly useful for cold applications and mainly used for the bottom part of the lining.

Most of the ramming mixes consist of refractory aggregates and semi-plastic bonding phase, which contains clay (conventionally) for the plastic property. The ramming mass gets kneaded when rammed under pressure, usually by pneumatic rammers. Various refractory aggregates, namely alumina, clay, magnesia, silica, and zircon are used as per the chemical requirement of the application area. As ramming process involves some external pressure and the composition is semidry in nature, contains less moisture, the rammed lining exhibits lower porosity and better density. Nearly no flowability or movement of the mass is required for installation. Hence, the particle sizes and their distribution for ramming masses are different than the castables. As flow is not important, so less liquid is used for the installation, the amount of fines is also reduced in the composition whereas the amount of intermediate fractions is high. Also, the grain compaction is achieved during the ramming process by external pressure. The major advantages of ramming masse are as follows:

1. Better compaction
2. Lesser liquid (water), so shorter drying period
3. Faster installation
4. Installation can be done at a higher temperature than castable and others

The binder system of the ramming mass is important and it depends on the application conditions. Binders may be of organic and inorganic in nature. Organic binders used are cellulose, lingo-sulfonate, molasses, etc. Also, coal tar, pitch, and resin are used as a binder for the systems containing non-oxide components, like carbon, as these binders can disperse carbon easily. Also they contain a higher amount of fixed carbon and impart carbon in the composition. Organic binders produce lower strength after the burnout of the binder's carbonaceous matter. After burnout or oxidation, a relatively porous structure is obtained, resulting in reduced hot strength and poor resistance to corrosion, oxidation, and abrasion. Among various inorganic binders, clay, phosphoric acid, phosphates, sol, and boric acid are important. Sol-bonded compositions have lower initial strength due to poor coagulation bonding but strength increases with an increase in temperature. Also, sol produces better heat strength.

Ramming is always done by vertical buildups of the material layer wise so the compaction of one layer is achieved first and then the next layer is rammed. As the ramming process cannot impart great force, thickness above 100–150 mm cannot transmit the pressure to the material below and so layer thickness is restricted. After each layer of the rammed mass, the surface needs to be scratched to enhance the bonding between the different layers to avoid laminations. This is due to lesser self-bonding character of ramming masses. The amount of liquid to be used is also important as a dry mass will not compact well due to less bonding and presence of excess liquid will make the material slide. In both the cases, poorly dense porous structure will be produced. The rammed lining needs to be dried carefully and slowly so that the surface does not get hard and impervious to the moisture vapor coming from the below layers; otherwise cracking will occur.

13.4.3 Gunning Mass

Gunning mass or gunite mix is another class of monolithic refractory, similar in composition and formulation to castable but with finer particle sizes. Use of gunning mass is a well-proven repair technique of refractory that can be applied quickly and cheaply. It is used for the hot repair of ladles and melting furnaces as well as relining or cold repair of the back-up lining. A refractory mass with different size fractions and additives is forced under pneumatic pressure and placed on the desired area, where the lining is to be done, using a special equipment having a mixer machine and a gun. There are two basic methods, namely, dry gunning and wet gunning.

In the dry gunning process, the dry composition of refractory is partially moistened with a part of the total water used, to reduce dusting and initiation of bond (cement) hydration. The dampened mix is then transported through a hose by pneumatic pressure. The hose is capable of withstanding relatively high temperature and is hung from the top of the kiln or furnace where the gunning lining is to be done. At the end of the hose is a nozzle assembly where water is mixed with the refractory stream and the resulting mixture is gunned onto the desired area. Initial dampening is done by about 5% of moisture and final mixing with water at the nozzle is done with about 5%–10% moisture. The position of the equipment may be adjusted with the help of a crane. A binocular may be used (for critical locations where a human cannot enter mainly due to high temperature) to identify the worn-out (corroded) area where repair is required, and then the equipment is placed in the proper direction and position for gunning. This method is highly dependent on the conveyance of the premixed mass.

In wet gunning technique, the refractory mass is moistened with the total required water in the mixer itself and then pumped through the hose using an eccentric screw or a piston pump. At the end of the hose, the material is dispersed with compressed air through the nozzle. For wet gunning, the machine or the hose may get clogged by the moistened refractory, particularly when the equipment is not in continuous use. Also, the equipment requires more intensive cleaning. With dry gunning system, the blockages in the conveying hose can be blown off easily by compressed air only.

The performance of the gunned lining is dependent on the refractory system used and the binder. The gunning (lining) thickness is typically maintained between 10 and 30 mm and can be used for operation after about 3–5 min of gunning. Standard gunning materials are made of magnesia, alumina, or silica base. Three essential requirements for a good gunning repair are optimal moistening, homogeneous mixing with water, and a high quality gunning machine that guarantees even conveying. Less moisture may result in higher dusting, fall of material, and poor property development and service life. The excessive moisture results in running off of the installed surface and poor performance. Also, higher water leads to clogging and hardening of the refractory mass within the hose, especially for the quick binding systems. Hence, gunning is a skilled activity and is dependent on the skill of the person.

Various bonding systems can be used for gunning materials. Alumina cement is useful for the low-temperature strength development. Again depending on the application temperatures, different amounts of cements are used for the gunning material. Phosphate bonding shows better bonding of gunning mass with the metallic surfaces. Resin bonding is used for the non-oxide-containing systems, especially for carbon and carbide-containing systems, like blast furnace trough. Colloidal silica is also a good binder for the gunning masses, and there is no degradation of strength at the intermediate temperatures. Sol bonding is also used for the blast furnace trough applications. Binder system may vary depending upon the installation temperature and final application temperature. For any bonding system, the target of gunning is to get a

1. Crack-free homogeneous lining

2. Minimum dust generation and rebound loss

3. Good adhesion of material with the development of high density and strength

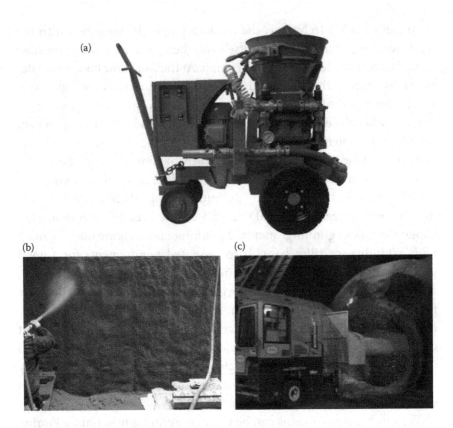

FIGURE 13.2   (a) Gunning machine, (b) gunning repair of reheating furnace, and (c) gunning operation in a steel converter (BOF).

Gunning is a very common repair technique mostly used in the iron and steel industries. It allows hot repair of the lining, making the whole process economic with reduced downtime. Gunning repair is common for blast furnace lining repair, trough areas, steel converter, steel ladle, and reheating furnaces. Figure 13.2 shows the gunning repair of steel converter (basic oxygen furnace) and reheating furnace.

13.4.4 Plastic Mass

The first patent on monolithic refractory was on plastic or pliable refractory in 1914, so this material can be taken as first developed unshaped refractory. Plastic mass is supplied in moldable, preformed blocks or slices in airtight condition and placed by pasting or ramming for a quick, economical, and emergency repair of the furnaces. Plastic mass can take any shape due to its plasticity and generally without any shuttering former for placement and installation. Depending on the thickness of the walls, the slice or block or its part, is broken off or cut out and placed (by pasting or ramming) into position. After installation, the plastic mass is levelled, and proper attention is required for the drying process, to avoid cracks and differential shrinkage, as the mass contains a higher amount of moisture or liquid. Also hard crust surface formation must be avoided during drying to avoid cracking or spalling of the lining. These materials can be both air-setting and heat-setting types, depending on the application requirements. Plastic mass, generally applied by hand pasting with a thin lining, is termed as a patching mass.

Plastic mass is made up of two main components, namely aggregate, like fireclay, bauxite, high alumina, and mullite and a bond that provides plasticity. Aggregate system is important for the final property development and decides the application area. Among bonding systems, the most common and oldest one is the plastic clay. It is widely used due to availability and cheap cost but is associated with high shrinkage due to moisture removal (dehydration of physically absorbed and chemically bonded water). Clay–sulfate bonds are also used due to its high strength and economic advantage. Most of the plastic masses are phosphate bonded. Phosphate bond sets slowly, keeps the mass workable for a prolonged time, and allows easy placement. Organic bonds like resin, coal tar, pitch, and molasses are also used but can leave carbon in the refractory mass, hence useful for compositions containing carbon or non-oxide components. The property of the plastic mass varies with the bond used. Generally, some deformable character of plastic refractory remains till it is not completely hard fired. This helps plastic refractory masses to have deformable character and a higher work of fracture. Hence, a plastic refractory resists the propagation of crack and crack growth in a better way. Also, it has a better thermal shock resistance property.

13.4.5 Spray Mass and Shotcrete

The spray mass composition and its application are very similar to gunning mass but with further reduced particle sizes. Generally, the maximum size used is 1 mm. This spray mass acts as a protective coating for the main lining and acts as the hot face refractory, facing all the abrasion, corrosion, and other effects. In spray technique, as the material is fine and spraying is done from a closer distance than gunning, the rebound loss and wastage of material is very minimum. Spraying can be done on a hot surface also.

The spray mass is applied by a specially designed spray machine in which water is mixed with dry composition and made into a free-flowing homogenous slurry. This fully wetted slurry is then pumped to the spray nozzle through a hose where it is atomised with air and sprayed effectively on the surface where the lining is to be done. The total spray machine consists of

1. A large hopper (capacity up to 3 ton of material)

2. A weighing system to precisely weigh the amount of material to mix

3. A mixer machine (sometimes with automatic control) that can provide kneading action also with the provision of water addition (with automatic control) to develop desired flowability and consistency

4. Pumping facility to push the mixed material with desired consistency through the hose pipe

5. A compressed air operated spray nozzle

The total amount of water used is about 15%–25% to impart flowing nature and spray ability in the dry material. After spraying the mass, heating of the lining is done on a predetermined schedule to remove the moisture first, and a slow schedule is maintained due to a higher amount of water present. Next the temperature is increased gradually to 600–700°C for complete water removal and spray mass lining becomes dry and hard. This spay mass does not sinter well with the main (permanent) lining due to its different particle characters and other properties. So a weak parting plane remains between the spay mass and the permanent lining that helps them to remove easily (deskulling) if required. Spray mass (MgO containing) is a common hot face lining for the tundish for steel industries, as shown in Figure 13.3a.

The main advantages of spray mass are as follows:

1. Only a few mm lining thickness is done to face the aggressive condition of the hot face

2. Minimum rebound loss

3. Less skull formation and easy deskulling

4. Flexibility to use in cold/hot condition

(a)   (b)

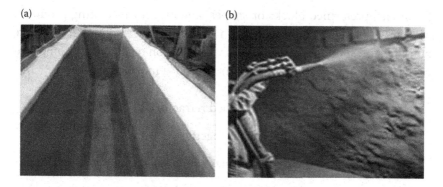

FIGURE 13.3 (a) Basic spray mass lined tundish and (b) shotcreting repair is in progress.

5. Less manpower is required

6. Can be applied either on shaped or unshaped permanent lining

Very similar to spray mass is a shotcrete mass where an additional liquid bonding or hardening agent is mixed with the pumped moistened mass at the nozzle mouth. Both setting accelerator and coagulating additives can be used to set the shotcrete faster. This technique was originally developed for the construction industries and has the advantages of high installation rate and good mechanical properties. Generally, a composition with self-flowing consistency is preferable for better pumpability and flow with low rebound loss. Shotcreteing on a permanent refractory lining is shown in Figure 13.3b.

Shotcrete is similar to gunning mass from technical and application points of view but is applied with a further developed technology. In shotcrete, the composition is premixed with water and a homogeneous mixture is obtained, which results in uniform properties all through the lining. Whereas, in gunning, water is added at the nozzle, hence less chance of homogenization that deteriorates the property of the lining. Again due to lack of homogenization and mixing, dust generation is high with greater rebound loss for gunning materials. Hence, shotcrete produces good lining with the uniform property, without any lamination and void structure.

13.4.6 Mortar

Mortars are used to fill refractory joints, bond refractory shapes together, and protect the joints from an attack of slag or other fluxes. They are used for bricks, preformed blocks or shapes, and also for insulating products. Mortars should be compatible with the main refractory that they are bonding and should not have excessive expansion or shrinkage compared to that lining material. The main functions of a mortar are

1. Filling of the gap between shaped refractories
2. Holding the individual shapes together
3. Retain the definite shape and size of the total lining
4. To prevent corrosive and abrasive attacks

The composition of these materials consists of fine aggregates and bond phase, which varies depending on the quality of the shape used and the field of application. The aggregate phase is similar to the shaped refractory material (sometimes the powdered form of the same refractory) to match the properties with them. The binder may be of inorganic or organic in nature; among inorganic bonds, clay, silicate, and phosphates are used and among organic bonds lignosulphonate, resin, and tar are common. These materials are delivered to the user industries either in a dry or a ready-to-use state. They are of two main types

1. Heat-setting mortar, which hardens at elevated temperatures by chemical or ceramic bonds
2. Air-setting mortar, which hardens at ambient temperature by chemical or hydraulic bonds

Mortars are porous and weaker in strength than the shaped refractories, for which they are used. This is due to higher moisture content in them. This porous structure makes them flexible and helps to accommodate the volumetric changes of the shaped refractory on temperature fluctuations and heating cooling cycles.

13.4.7 Dry Vibratable Mass

Dry vibratable mass (DVM) is a special unshaped refractory where no liquid or water is required for placement and installation. It is also a hot face refractory lining, which acts as a coating on a permanent lining and faces all the stringent conditions of the hot face, similar to spray mass. This was developed in the 1980s, close to the development of the spraying mass for the iron and steel industries, but did not become popular due to its relatively higher cost and environmental issues.

The main advantages of DVM are as follows:

1. Easy installation as no mixing process is required with water

2. Faster drying period as no moisture removal

3. Economic as it saves fuel

4. No drying defects

5. No hydrogen pickup (for molten steel during casting)

6. No direct adhesion with the permanent lining and easy deskulling

7. Longer service life

8. Free flowing in nature, helping the installation process and equipment simpler and easier

DVM can be of both hot setting and cold setting types. For cold set system, dry powder is mixed with a liquid binder and hardener in a screw feeder before installation. Mixing of the additives is critical for the final performance of the lining. The hot set materials are more flexible and user-friendly. Dry material is directly poured in the area of lining using the former. During installation, vibration is done for better filling and compaction of DVM. After installation, the lining is cured with the former in place. The most common heating method is to use hot air blowing system using natural gas or LPG as the fuel. DVM lining also helps in reducing the energy cost. After the specific curing schedule, the former is removed, and the refractory lining is ready for operation.

The bond system plays the major role in the installation and performance of these materials. Initial development was started with phenolic resin, but disadvantages like low installation temperature, use of a parting agent for smooth former separation, the evolution of harmful gases, and cost are associated with it. Commercially available sodium silicate is also used, but demerits like low strength and the high sodium level potentially affect its performance. Abundantly available cheap glucose ($C_6H_{12}O_6$) is being used widely due to its advantages like thermoplastic nature, allowing the lining to install even above 300°C, economy, and environmental friendliness. The most common application of DVM is in the tundish hot face lining, as shown in Figure 13.4.

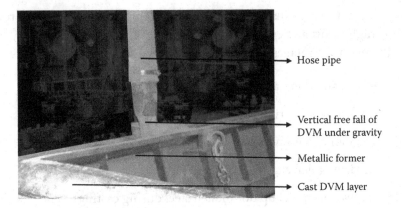

Hose pipe

Vertical free fall of
DVM under gravity

Metallic former

Cast DVM layer

FIGURE 13.4   DVM lining of tundish is in operation.

13.5 MAIN APPLICATION AREAS

Castable with varying alumina content are important for tundish safety lining, VAD and VOD covers, snorkel of RH unit of secondary steel making, DRI (sponge iron) making rotary kilns, reheating furnaces, blast furnace tuyeres, preheaters of cement rotary kilns, boilers, incinerators, annealing and heat treatment furnaces, soaking pits, aluminum melting, and holding furnaces. Precast shapes of castables are used in ladle bottoms, burner block, dam and weir of the tundish, electric arc furnace spout and delta regions, well block, and seating block of steel ladles. Very high alumina (>98%) containing castables are used in carbon black reactor, coal gasifiers, and petrochemical industries. Alumina–spinel based castables are used in steel ladle, seating and well blocks of ladles, porous plug, electric arc furnace delta and launder, tundish dams, and weirs. Alumina–silicon carbide–carbon-based castables, both with cement and sol bonding, are used in the blast furnace trough lining.

High alumina–based plastic masses are useful for silver melting furnaces and acid regeneration plants. Alumina–silicon carbide–carbon-based plastic mass is useful for blast furnace tap hole. Alumina-based ramming mass and plastic mass are important for the repair work of EAF launders, petrochemical industries, and hydrocarbon industries. Insulating castable containing alumina from 15 to 50 wt% are useful for petrochemical industries, especially as backup lining, heater, stack, and the duct of petroleum reformer and also in hydrocarbon process industries.

Silica-based ramming masses are important for the lining of the cupola of iron and steel industries, coke ovens, and coreless induction furnaces. Silica-based spray mass are used for hot repair of coke oven walls.

MgO-based basic ramming and gunning mass are used for the repair of steelmaking electric arc furnaces, induction furnaces, steel converters (BOF), ladles, hot metal mixers, RH degasser, etc. MgO-based basic spray mass and dry vibrating masses are used widely for tundish hot face lining. Dolomite-based basic ramming and gunning masses are used in AOD vessel, ladle furnace, electric arc furnace, and steelmaking converters.

13.6 SUMMARY

Refractory materials that are supplied from the manufacturers' end without any shape are termed as unshaped or monolithic refractories. These loose dry materials are usually mixed with liquid (commonly water) at the user site and then applied. Unshaped refractories have many advantages over shaped refractories and replace the shaped refractories in most of the industrial applications.

There are different ways of classifying unshaped refractories and among them, classification based on application (installation) technique is most widely accepted and used. These are castable, ramming mass, gunning mass, plastics, and spray mass.

Other than the conventional raw materials used for making shaped refractories, unshaped ones require some special materials. Property-modified fine fractions are important to control the matrix phase. Bonding materials are used to develop strength after shaping and also to enhance sintering. Property-enhancing additives are required, especially for the cement-containing compositions, like silica fume, dispersants, antisetting agents, and different fibers.

Various unshaped refractories are used in various industrial applications. Mostly they replace the shaped refractories in all the different applications.

QUESTIONS AND ASSIGNMENTS

1. What is unshaped refractory? What are the advantages?

2. What are the different types of unshaped refractories used industrially?

3. Why do we need bonding material in unshaped refractory?

4. What are the different bonding materials used for unshaped refractory?

5. What is the difference between building cement and refractory cement?

6. Describe the hydration mechanism of calcium aluminate cement.

7. Why developmental work continues to replace cement in the unshaped refractory?

8. What are the advantages of silica sol as a refractory binder?

9. How does a silica sol help in the development of strength?

10. How does a phosphate bond work in the unshaped refractory?

11. What is a hydratable alumina? Explain its hydration mechanism.

12. Compare the different bonding systems used for unshaped refractories.

13. What is silica fume and how does it improve the properties of castables?

14. What are the functions of dispersant and antisetting agent?

15. How does an organic fiber help? What is the role of a metallic fiber?

16. Write in detail on castables.

17. Compare ramming mass and gunning mass of an unshaped refractory.

18. What is a plastic refractory? How does it work?

19. Write in detail about spray mass and dry vibratable mass.

20. Write about the different applications of unshaped refractories.

BIBLIOGRAPHY

1. ISO 1927: Refractory products: prepared unshaped dense and insulating materials classification.
2. C. Parr and Ch. Wohrmeyer, The advantages of calcium alumina cement as a castable bonding system, *St. Louis Section meeting of American Ceramic Society*, St. Louis, MN, 2006.
3. B. Nagai, Recent advances in castable refractories, *Taikabutsu Refractories*, 9(1), 2–9, 1987.

4. T. A. Bier, N. E. Bunt, and C. Parr, Calcium aluminate bonded castables: Their advantages and applications, *Proc. The 25th Annual Meeting of the Association of Latin-American Refractory Manufacturers (ALAFAR)*, vol. I, pp. 75–84, December 1–4, Bariloche, Argentina, 1996.

5. K. M. Parker and J. H. Sharp, Refractory calcium aluminate cement, *Transactions Journal British Ceramic Society*, 81, 35–42, 1982.

6. W. E. Lee, W. Vieira, S. Zhang, K. G. Ahari, H. Sarpoolaky, and C. Parr, Castable refractory concrete, *International Materials Reviews*, 46(3), 145–167, 2001.

7. S. Banerjee, *Monolithic Refractories—A Comprehensive Handbook*, World Scientific/The American Ceramic Society, Singapore, 311p, 1998.

8. S. Banerjee, Recent developments in monolithic refractories, *American Ceramic Society Bulletin*, 77(10), 59–63, 1998.

9. Y. Hongo, ρ-alumina bonded castable refractories, *Taikabutsu Overseas*, 9 (1), 35–38, 1988.

10. R. Racher, Improved workability of calcia free alumina binder alpha bond for non-cement castables, *Presented at the 9th Biennial Worldwide Congress on Refractories*, November 8–11, Orlando, FL, 2005.

11. W. Ma and P. W. Brown, Mechanisms of the reaction of hydratable aluminas, *Journal of the American Ceramic Society*, 82(2), 453–456, 1999.

12. R. K. Iler, *The Chemistry of Silica: Solubility, Polymerization, Colloid and Surface Properties and Biochemistry*, New York, Wiley, 866p, 1979.

13. S. Banerjee, Versatility of gel bond castable/pumpable refractories, *Refractories Applications and News*, 6(1), 1–3, 2001.

14. W. E. Lee, W. Vieira, S. Zhang, K. Ghanbari Ahari, H. Sarpoolaky, and C. Parr, Castable refractory concretes, *International Materials Review*, 46(3), 145–167, 2001.

15. J. E. Cassidy, Phosphate bonding then and now, *American Ceramic Society Bulletin*, 56(7), 640–643, 1977.

16. R. Giskow, J. Lind and E. Schmidt, The variety of phosphates for refractory and technical applications by the example of aluminium phosphates, *Ceramic Forum International*, 81, E1–E5, 2004.

17. S. K. Das, R. Sarkar, P. Mondal, and S. Mukherjee, No cement high alumina self flow castable, *American Ceramic Society Bulletin*, 82(2), 55–59, 2003.

18. R. Sarkar, S. K. Das, P. K. Mandal, S. N. Mukherjee, S. Dasgupta, and S. K. Das, Fibre reinforced no cement self flow high alumina castable—A study, *Transactions of the Indian Ceramic Society*, 62(1), 1–4, 2003.

19. R. Sarkar, S. Mukherjee, and A. Ghosh, Gel bonded Al2O3–SiC–C based blast furnace trough castable, *American Ceramic Society Bulletin*, 85(5), 9101–9105, 2006.

20. A. K. Singh and R. Sarkar, Effect of binders and distribution coefficient on the properties of high alumina castables, *Journal of the Australian Ceramics Society*, 50(2), 93–98, 2014.

21. R. Sarkar, A. Kumar, S. P. Das, and B. Prasad, Silica sol bonded high alumina castable: Effect of reduced sol, *Refractories World Forum*, 7(2), 83–87, 2015.

22. R. Sarkar and A. Parija, Effect of alumina fines on vibratable high alumina low cement castable, *Interceram*, 63(3), 113–116, 2014.

23. R. Sarkar and A. Satpathy, High alumina self flow castable with different binders, *Refractories World Forum*, 4(4), 98–102, 2012.

24. R. Sarkar and A. Mishra, High alumina self flow castable with different cement binders, *Refractories Manual*, 107–111, 2012.

25. R. Sarkar and A. Parija, Effect of alumina fines on high alumina self-flow low cement castables, *Refractories World Forum*, 6(1), 73–77, 2014.

26. R. Sarkar and S. K. Das, Effect of distribution coefficient on gel bonded high alumina castable, *IRMA Journal*, 43(1), 31–36, 2010.

27. J. B. Johnson and K. J. Saylor, A comparison of disposable magnesite tundish lining systems. *73rd ISS Steel Making Conference*, Detroit, MI, 1990.

28. M. J. Bradley, Overview of tundish dry vibe technology, *MPT International*, 2, 70–72, 2008.

29. M. W. Vance and K. J. Moody, Steel plant refractories containing alpha bond hydratable alumina binders, *Alcoa Technical Bulletin,* Alcoa Industrial Chemicals, Pittsburgh, PA, 1996.

30. P. Tassot, Cold setting DVM for tundish a real alternative. *Proceedings of the 3rd Int. Conf. on Refractories at Jamshedpur,* pp. 187–191, India (ICRJ), 2013.

Index

Printed in the United States
by Baker & Taylor Publisher Services